100 DAYS OF HERBS

Small daily tasks to cultivate a deeper
connection with herbal practices

Jessica Marcy

Founder of Old Wisdom Wellness
& Sweet Love & Ginger

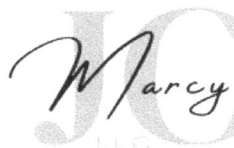

First edition June 2023

Book Design by Jessica Marcy
Book Photos by Jessica Marcy & Rachel McNair

Paperback ISBN: 9798988406600

ebook ISBN: 9798988406617

Published by JC Marcy LLC DBA Old Wisdom Wellness
www.oldwisdomwellness.com

For Eric, whose steadfast
support and love made
all of this possible.

TABLE OF CONTENTS

TABLE OF CONTENTS CONTINUED

Introduction

The first question I am often asked after a class, or discussion about herbs is, "How do I get started?" It is a question that plagues herbalists all over. How do we explain to these inquisitive souls that each and every herbal journey is different? That the path that led us to where we are, will not be the same as what leads them? How do we distill down years of study, and experimentation to a handful of simple actions that will actually guide these people in a helpful direction?

I began by suggesting books, blogs, and websites that I have personally learned from over the years, but so often I don't know the person to whom I'm speaking with and later learning that my suggestions were either over or underwhelming for them. When I began teaching classes, both in person and online, I found the information I wanted to impart was overwhelming, and that writing workbooks for said classes would only go so far.

The image of this book began to take shape in my mind over these various conversations and experiences. I wanted to bring together the idea that herbs can be a part of everyday life, without being all-encompassing or overwhelming. Years of experience aren't required for simple preparations, and herbs aren't as unreliable as many of us are led to believe. Humans have been using herbs as medicine since the dawn of our time with every pocket of human culture on this planet has seen the use of herbs. We now have archeological evidence going as far back as 60,000 years showing the use of medicinal plants. In modern day, the use of herbs as medicine is considered "alternative" and unfortunately they're often received with skepticism. It is my quest to change that perception and to show that herbs and herbal medicine can be a beautiful part of any lifestyle. Most of all, I wanted to make the use of herbs at home - accessible to everyone.

This book is a collection of tasks that can mostly be completed in an hour or less of devoted time each day. Some tasks may require longer cooking/drying/soaking times, but the dedicated and focused time is much less. When added together, these small tasks can show the power of even basic herbal knowledge as well as how to integrate that knowledge into daily life.

While there is a table of contents at the beginning of the book that outlines each task of the 100 day journey, there are also two indexes at the back of the book that my be of greater use. These allow the reader to search by herb, as well as preparation; allowing the reader to focus on a specific herb or perfect a certain preparation should they choose. While the obvious objective of this book is to have the reader move through in chronological order, it is also encouraged to group tasks as may be required or preferred. For example, when a specific herb such as lemon balm is in season, it would be in the reader's best interest to prepare all the recipes that utilize that herb before its season has passed. It's also possible that some days are busier than others, and the reader may choose to group tasks simply because they have the available time.

Everyone's path to learning how to use herbs is as unique as they are. Please feel free to experiment; not only with the plants themselves, but with this book and its preparations.

Additional resources and downloadable worksheet pages can be found at www.oldwisdomwellness.com/100daysdownloads.

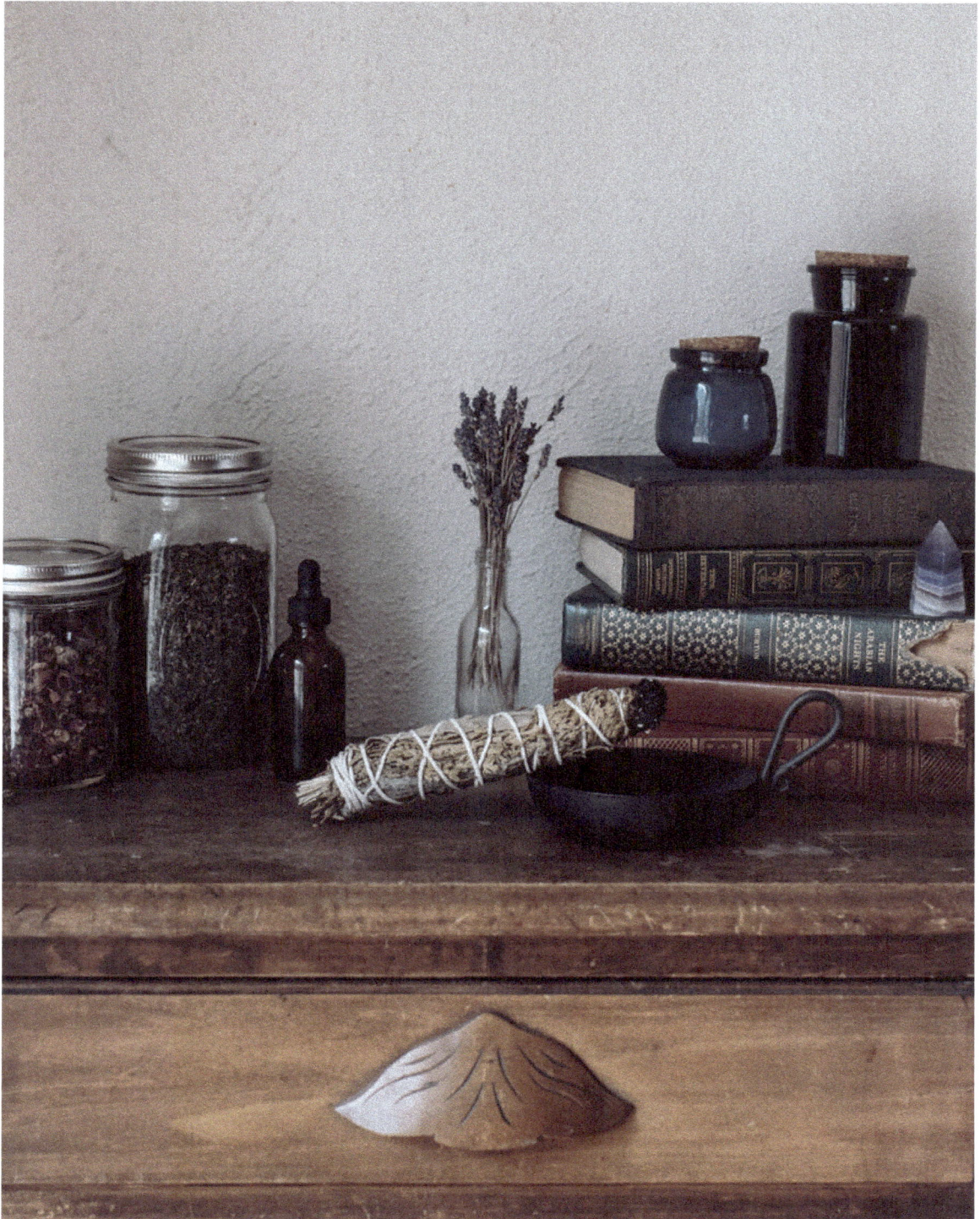

Make a Cup of Herbal Tea

Herbal teas or infusions are often most people's first introduction to working with herbs. To begin the 100-day journey of working with herbs by brewing a simple cup of tea seems appropriate. Choose a single dried herb for your cup of tea. Take your time; smell and touch the herb before it steeps.

To make a cup of loose leaf tea, measure 1-2 tsps of dried herb into a tea strainer and place it in a mug. Pour 8-10 oz of hot water over the tea and let it steep as desired. Remove the strainer with the herbs and discard.

Once steeped, smell it again. How it is different? What about the taste? Is it what you expected? Drink slowly, and see how the flavor changes over time.

Reflect on how you feel during and after enjoying your cup. Are these feelings expected with this herb? Record your thoughts here:

Gather your Tools

There are not many things needed to begin your herbal journey, but a few good things to have on hand include:

Jars (various sizes) with sealable tops
Unbleached wax paper for lining lids
Cheesecloth
Fine mesh strainer
Double boiler (or improvised one)
Measuring spoons & cups
Whisk
Tea strainer (smaller than the fine mesh strainer)
Mugs/tea cups
Pots and pans of varying sizes
Masking tape & pens for labels

In addition to gathering tools, it is important to source high quality dried herbs, especially if you have plans to use them medicinally. Some may be lucky enough to have a local herb shop or farm, but for most, sourcing herbs will be done via the internet. Places like Mountain Rose Herbs, Frontier Co-op, Davids Organic, and Starwest Botanicals are all great options for purchasing dried herbs.

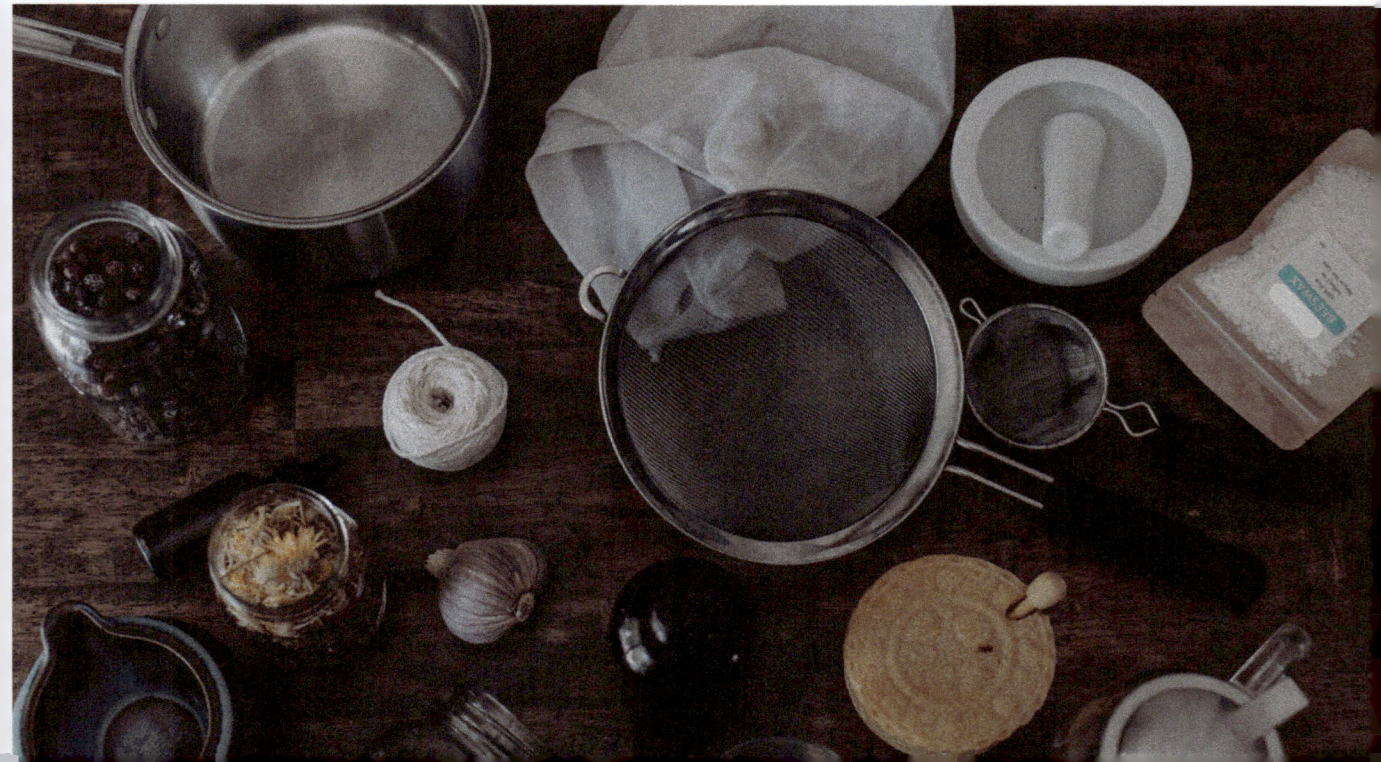

Kitchen Herbcraft

Look through your kitchen cabinets and take stock of the herbs that you have on hand. Many culinary herbs have a long histories of medicinal use as well. Below are a few favored kitchen herbs and some of their medicinal uses:

Oregano (Origanum vulgare) Is commonly used for it's anti-bacterial, anti-fungal and anti-viral properties. It is also anti-inflammatory, high in antioxidants, and known to be beneficial for digestive health.

Thyme (Thymus vulgaris) As both an anti-spasmodic and an expectorant, thyme is beneficial for calming a cough while also helping to clear mucus from the lungs. Additionally, it is anti-bacterial, anti-viral, and anti-fungal.

Garlic (Allium sativum) One of the most popular herbs in the world, garlic has a reputation for bringing flavor, boosting immune function, reducing blood pressure, improving cholesterol, and even improving longevity. It is also anti-microbial, anti-fungal, and anti-parasitic; making it a great multipurpose herb.

Make a list of 2-3 of the kitchen herbs that you use the most, and research their medicinal uses. Use this space to take note of how you might like to try to utilize them medicinally in the future:

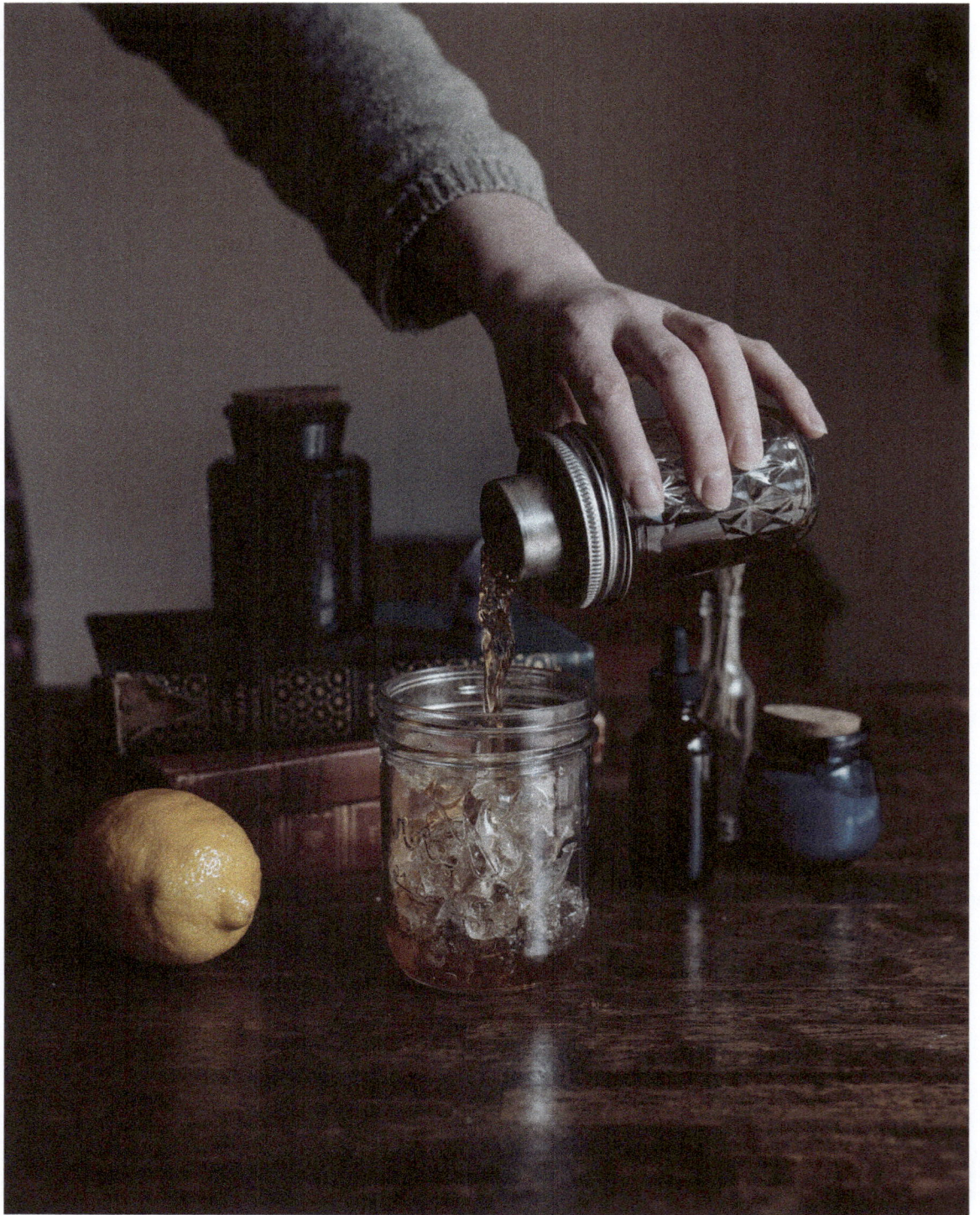

Lemon Balm Simple Syrup

Simple syrups are delicious and versatile preparations. In addition to being used medicinally, they can also be used for flavoring both food and beverage. Adding a simple syrup to a marinade, to top a dessert, or flavor sparkling water are just a few of the options.

When making herbal syrups, we typically strive for a 1:1 ratio by volume of honey or sugar to liquid herbal infusion. This ratio allows for a longer-lasting product (about 4 weeks in the fridge). However, if that is too sweet or you plan to use the syrup in 2 weeks or less, you can alter to a 2:1 ratio of 2 parts liquid herbal infusion to 1 part honey or sugar sweetener.

This recipe utilizes lemon balm (Melissa officinalis) for its many attributes. Not only has a lovely, mild flavor, but it is also a powerhouse when it comes to cold, flu, and virus care. It is anti-inflammatory, anti-viral, antiseptic, carminative, mildly sedative, and calming. It can be used to help with an upset or anxious stomach, for calming a fever, and fighting a viral condition making it a great choice for a simple syrup for kids.

In addition to it's medicinal capabilities, lemon balm has a long history of use for boosting spirits and calming nervous energy, especially those with a nervous stomach. A simple drink made of the syrup and seltzer can be a welcome evening treat after a long day, or to soothe an upset tummy. Simply combine 1 oz of the syrup with 6 oz of seltzer or water and top with ice. Add a lemon for garnish and to enhance the lemon flavor of the herb.

While making your syrup, take note of the scent of the herb and the way it changes the color of the syrup. Try comparing the flavor of the syrup to a tea made with lemon balm and note its differences.

Basic Herbal Simple Syrup

2 cups water
1-2 cups honey or sugar
½ cup dried herb

Combine water and sugar in a small pan. Bring to a simmer and stir until the sugar is completely dissolved, and the liquid is clear again.

Remove from heat and add the dried herbs. Cover and let stand for 20 minutes to 4 hours.

Strain and store refrigerated, in an airtight container for 1-2 weeks (2:1) or 3-4 weeks (1:1).

Use as desired.

05

Get in Touch with Herbs

Take some time and visit a local greenhouse or plant nursery. Take a look at the different herbs available. Smell them, touch them (carefully), take note of what is annual, perennial, and what grows well in your area.

While browsing the herb section, and really take a look at the plants; note their differences and similarities, their scent and texture. Which plants are similar? What makes them similar? Do any of the labels have the plants' scientific names?

Take note of some of the plant varieties and their names. For example; different varieties of mint all begin with Mentha for their scientific name, but the second word typically describes that varieties attributes. Peppermint has the scientific name, Mentha x piperita, while water mints scientific name is Mentha aquatica.

Consider purchasing an herb to grow at home. Many herbs can easily grow in a sunny window with little needs.

Some low maintenance herbs that are good for indoor gardens include: basil, parsely, mint, bay laurel, lemon balm, thyme, chives, tulsi, oregano, sage, rosemary, aloe, and catnip.

Already have a garden? Take some time to research the plants that you grow. Many ornamental plants also have medicinal qualities, such as feverfew, bee balm, lavender, marigold, fuchsia, chives, California poppy, as well as some varieties of violets, and hibiscus.

06

Compare Fresh vs Dried

Make 2 cups of tea; one with fresh herb, and the other with the same dried herb. Take your time and note the differences in scent and texture before and after steeping. What is different about the color, taste, and scent in the fresh vs dried teas? Write down your thoughts below:

What is a Menstruum?

A menstruum is a solvent or liquid that is used to dissolve or suspend extracts from plants. These can include but are not limited to alcohol (tinctures), oil, vinegar, glycerite, honey, or water infusions.

Each type of menstruum has different properties, and therefore the resulting extract is also different for each type of menstruum. For example, oil-based menstruums are better at extracting fat-soluble vitamins due to their high-fat content. Learn more about oil-based menstruums on day 12.

Menstruums that have a high water content are better at extracting high mineral plants such as nettle, red raspberry leaf, or alfalfa. These are usually in the form of teas or infusions, such as the nourishing herbal infusion made on days 19 & 20.

Alcohol-based menstruums tend to have an affinity for extracting pungent, bitter, and resinous herbs. When working with alcohol, it is important to pay attention to the alcohol strength and the plant material. Typically, lighter plant matter like leaves and flowers will require a lower proof alcohol to extract them, while more fibrous material such as roots, and bark will require a higher proof. Similarly, a higher proof is needed when extracting fresh plant material as opposed to dry due to the water content already contained in the fresh plant. This information can typically be found in most herbal references. See day 32 and the reference books on day 100 for further reading on these.

Vegetable glycerin is an odorless, viscous, sweet, liquid that is often used as a menstruum for aromatic, pungent, astringent, and sour herbs. While glycerin is chemically an alcohol, it is not processed in the body the same way and is often used as a replacement for those who avoid alcohol use - and for children. Additionally, it is low on the glycemic index and despite being sweet to the taste, is safe for those with diabetes or other blood sugar issues. Learn more about glycerites on day 64.

Similarly to alcohol and glycerin, vinegar is also a great menstruum for extracting aromatic, pungent, and bitter herbs. It is beneficial for culinary applications, anti-glycemic effects, and gut health. Unfortunately, using vinegar will not be as potent as using alcohol or glycerin, and will therefore require a higher dosage. This can be difficult, due to the overpowering flavor of many vinegars.

Note for infusing menstruums: some menstruums, like alcohol and vinegar, can be very corroding to metal lids. This is why it is important to line these types of lids with unbleached wax or parchment paper. This will also protect your infusion from the leaching of unwanted chemicals from plastic lids or lined metal lids.

08

Make a Bath Salt for Sore Muscles

It's well known that hot baths are a great way to relax after a long day, but they can also be beneficial to your physical health too. By adding herbs and other natural ingredients, it's possible to create a bath that can help the body detox, relieve pain, heal wounds, aid in muscle recovery, and more.

Herbs that are typically good for sore muscles are those that will increase circulation, decrease inflammation, and help in moving lymph fluid. These include mint, ginger, comfrey, rose, lavender, chamomile, rosemary, wintergreen, clove, and eucalyptus.

Sore Muscle Bath Soak

1/2 cup Epsom salt
1/2 cup baking soda
1/4 cup dried herbs
1 Tbsp castile soap
10 drops mild essential oils such as lavender, or chamomile

Combine Epsom salt, baking soda and herbs in a bowl.

Pour castile soap into a tablespoon and add the essential oils directly to the soap before adding to the bowl.

Stir all the ingredients together and add to a warm bath.

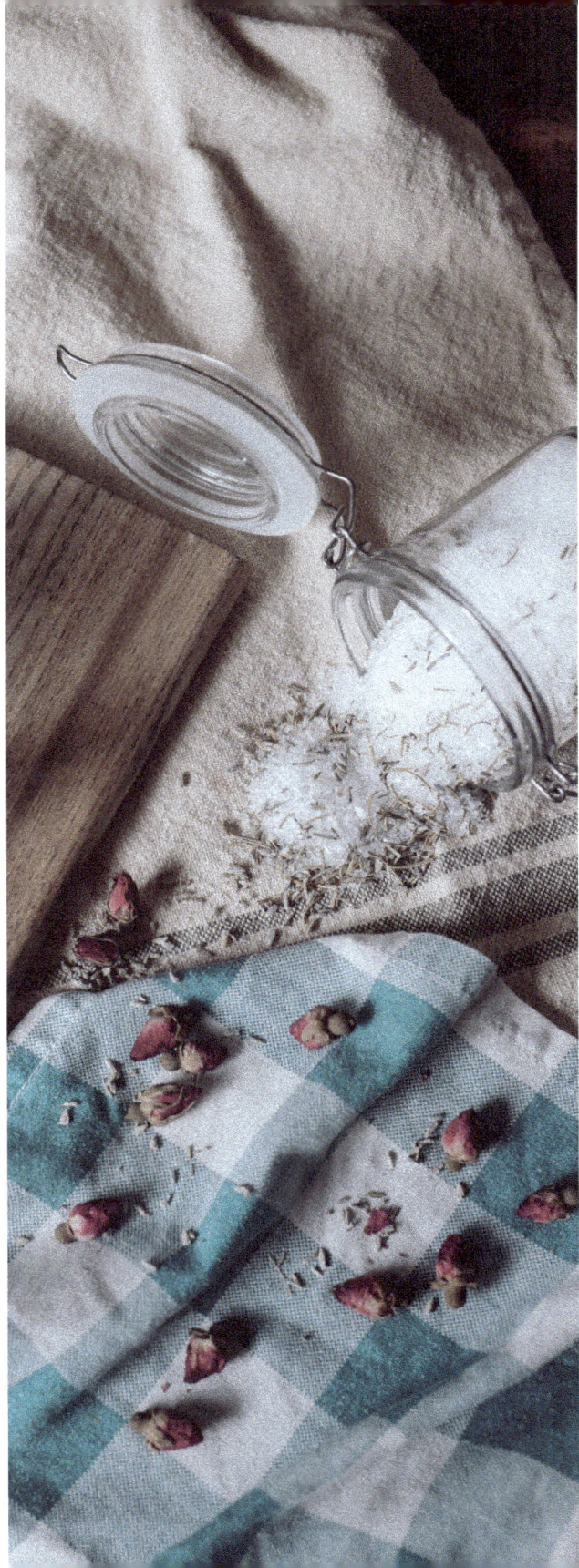

Culinary vs Medicinal

One of the first and most difficult lessons in learning herbalism is understanding how to utilize herbs medicinally versus culinary. Because herbs are perceived as natural, they are often misconstrued as safe at any and all levels. However, it is important to understand that anything natural or otherwise if used incorrectly can be harmful.

Many of us understand that using herbs and spices in our day-to-day cooking does not signify enough exposure to any one herb to result in a medicinal benefit. However, it is important to also view these as microdoses that can add up over time to create a medicinal dose. For example, drinking the same herbal tea every day for several weeks can often add up to a medicinal dose as the herbs build up in the system. Similarly, any herb eaten in meals multiple times a day – for several days – can also be considered medicinal. In some cultures, an herb can be eaten daily starting at a young age, in which case the body can build up a tolerance and become a culinary dose for that person. Should they choose to use the herb medicinally, they may require a larger dosage than others. For example, drinking the same herbal tea every day for several weeks can often add up to a medicinal dose, as the herbs build up in the system.

While this shows how subjective dosing can be from person to person, please keep in mind that more is not, in fact, always better. All herbal preparations have different strengths based not solely on their type of preparation, but on the volume of the herb used, the conditions it was grown in, and the potency at the time of extraction. Many times, overuse of an herbal preparation can cause an exacerbation of symptoms. In the example of herbs that are meant to support and nourish the system, if used too frequently, they can cause dehydration or diarrhea.

As a rule of thumb, it is suggested to first adhere to the recommended dosing on the container of any pre-bought herb. If the preparation is handmade, refer to appropriate source material for each herb in the preparation. For a preparation of many herbs, review the dosage suggestions for each herb and choose a dose that does not allow for overuse of any one herb in the blend. A list of books that can be used as source material is listed on day 100, as well as many preparations within have their dosage listed.

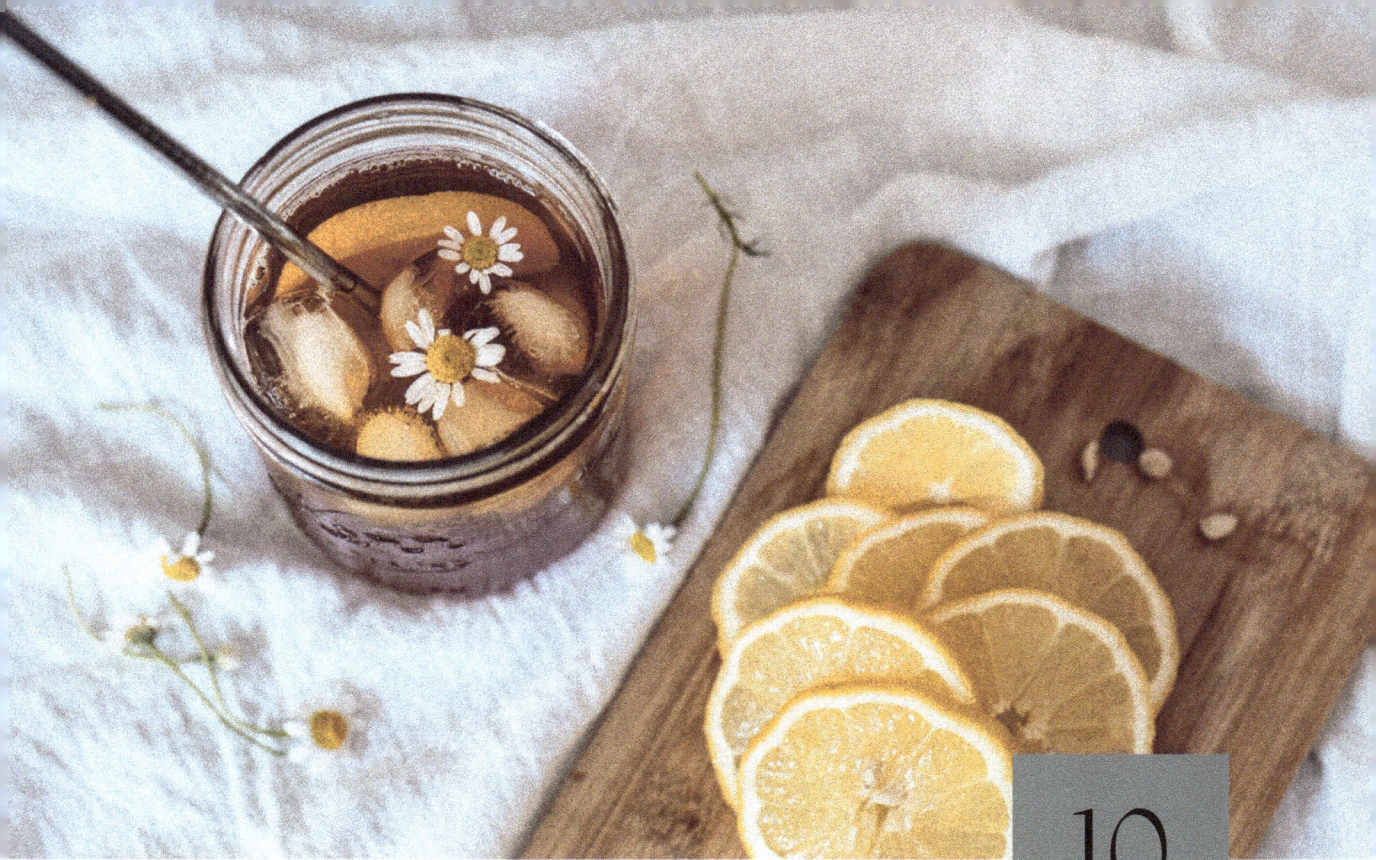

Iced Tea 3 Ways

Pour over method

1-2 tsp tea
1 cup hot water
Combine tea and water and let steep while covered for 4-8 minutes, to produce a strong-brewed tea. Strain and pour over ice. Serve immediately.

Cold Brewed

2-3 tsp tea
1 cup cold water
Combine tea and water and let steep, covered in the fridge for 8-12 hours. Strain and serve as desired.

Sun Tea

2-3 tsp tea
1 cup room temperature water
Combine tea and water, and cover. Place in direct sunlight and let steep, for 4-6 hours. Strain and serve as desired.

11

Make a Stress Relieving Oxymel

Drinking vinegars have been around for hundreds of years as a way to either make drinking water safe or to preserve fruit and herbs. In modern day, they can be used as refreshing herbal mocktails, salad dressings, marinades, and more. The benefits of adding drinking vinegar to your diet not only include the nutrients from the infusions you choose but also the probiotic and blood sugar balancing benefits of raw vinegar.

Oxymels are drinking vinegars that are created by soaking plant matter in vinegar and honey for 4-6 weeks. Shrubs are a variation of drinking vinegar that uses sugar instead of traditional honey and are sometimes made with the addition of heat. Switchels are yet another variation that combines vinegar, ginger, and molasses.

The recipe below is a traditional oxymel that contains not only the calming, nutrient-dense power of tulsi (Ocimum tenuiflorum) but also the sweet, antioxidant, electrolyte power of hibiscus (Hibiscus sabdariffa). While it is not needed, the option to add fruit such as lemon, orange, or berries would be a tasty addition.

While making this recipe, take note of the mixture as it steeps. See how the color changes as the ingredients meld together.

We will decant and use the final product on day 33.

Tulsi Hibiscus Oxymel

3/4 cup dried holy basil (tulsi) leaves
2 Tbsp dried hibiscus
1/3 cup honey
1 cup apple cider vinegar

Combine herbs in a clean jar.

Pour in apple cider vinegar, followed by the honey.

Seal with a glass, plastic or metal lid lined with parchment. Shake well and place in a cool dark place. Shake daily for roughly 2-4 weeks.

You may need to add more vinegar after the first 24 hours, to be sure the herbs are completely covered in liquid.

Once steeped, strain well and store in the fridge for up to 6 months. Discard if mold develops.

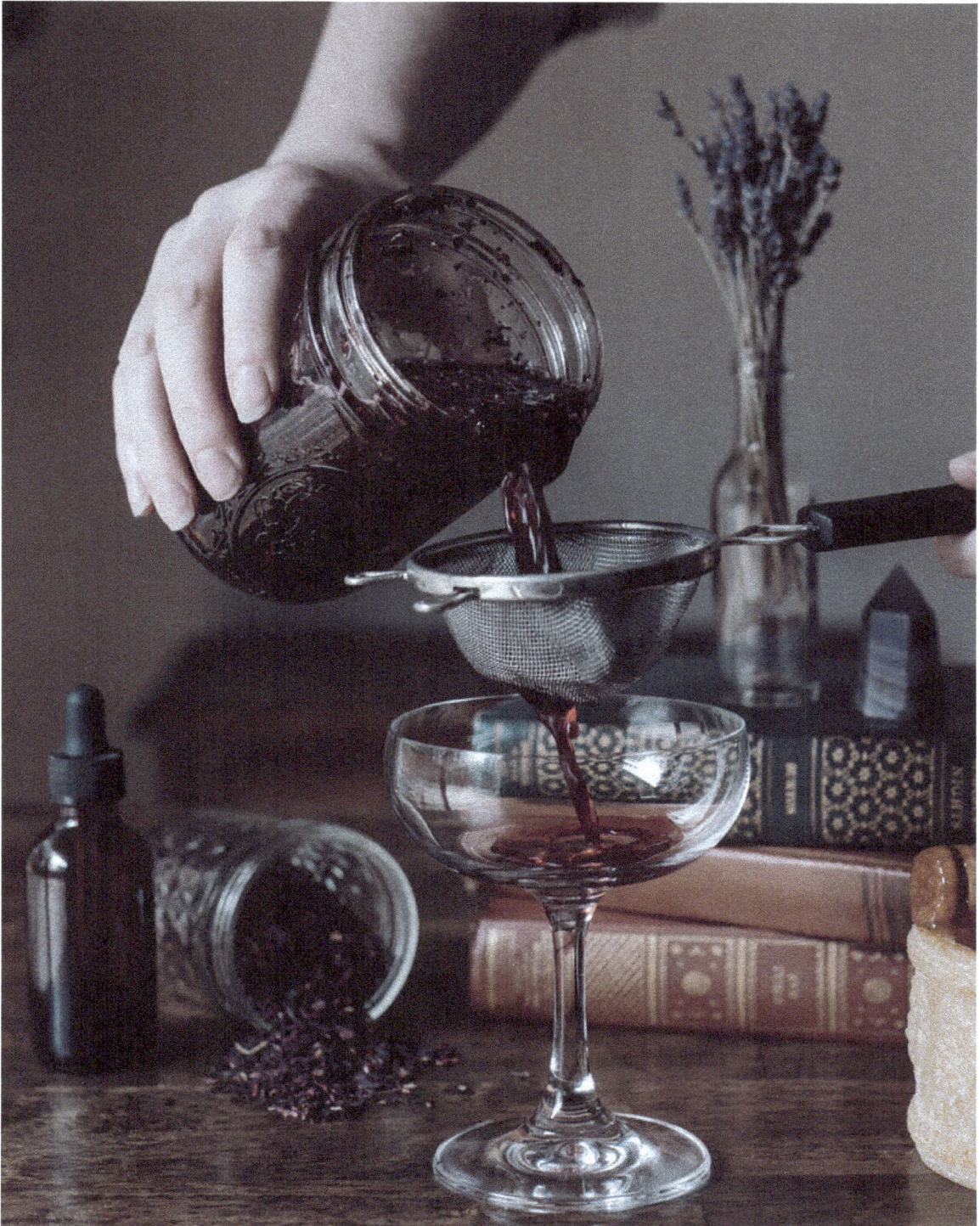

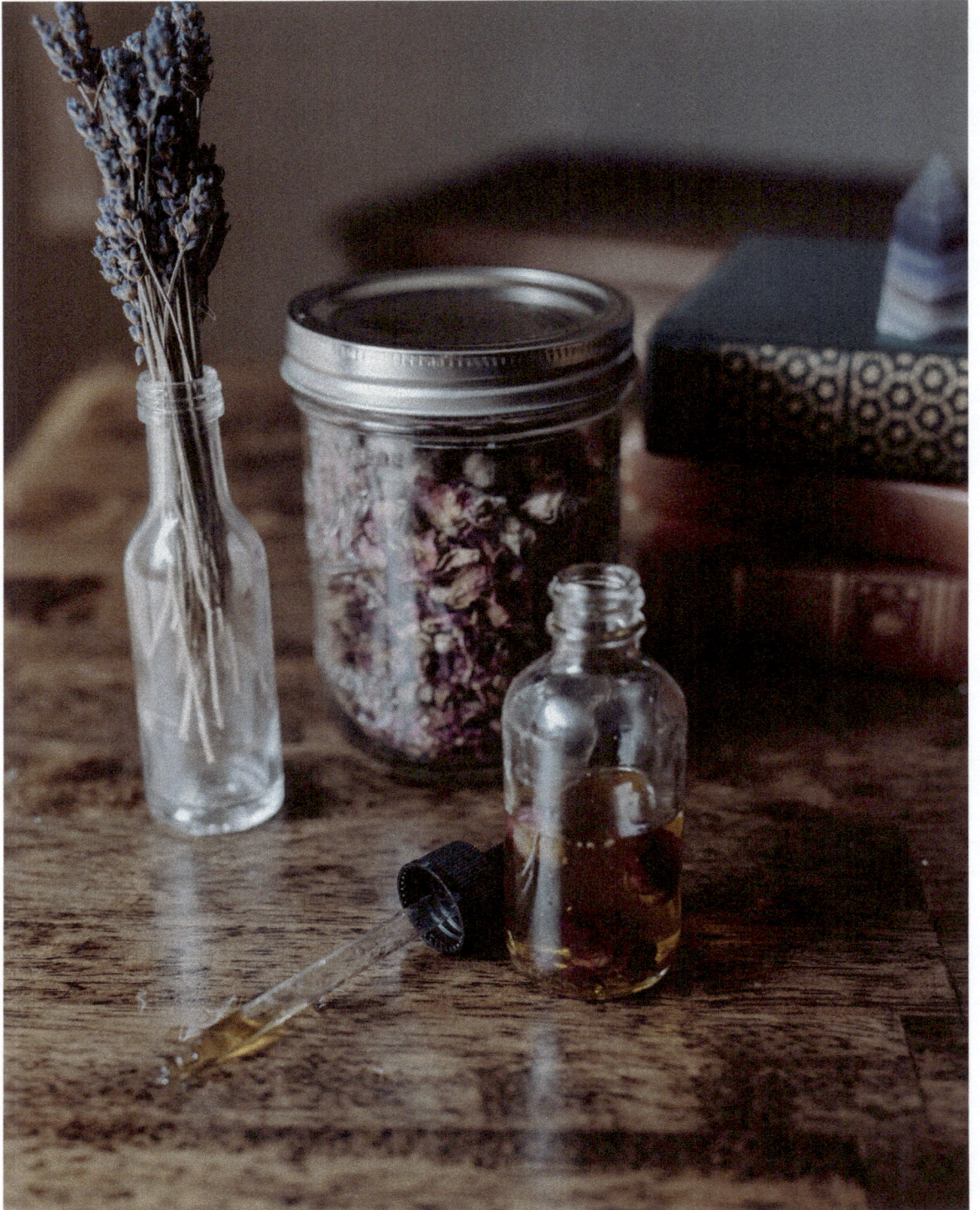

How to Choose
Oils for Extracting

Oil-based extracts are great for use both internally and externally. While they are not as potent as extracts such as alcohol or glycerin, they can still be used medicinally, especially for topical issues. Oils are great at extracting oil or fat-based vitamins from herbs (including essential oils and resins). Because of their gentle nature, most oils are generally considered safe for everyone including weak, elderly, and small children.

When considering what oils to use as a menstruum, it is important to also look at the properties of the oil itself and make sure it is in alignment with the goal of the extract. There are numerous uses for infused oils, such as topically, in beauty products and serums, internally, for cooking, flavoring, and administering medicine. Below is a list of some of the most commonly used oils for extraction.

Grapeseed Oil
Favored for its lightweight feel, grapeseed oil is high in vitamin E and easily absorbed into the skin. It can help with the effects of aging, and is widely accessible.

Coconut
Typically used for massage oils and skincare preparations, as it contains skin-nourishing fatty acids and polyphenols.

Olive Oil
One of the most used oils for it's long shelf life, olive oil is packed with fatty acids and plant sterols, making it great for cleansing and moisturizing dry skin. It is used in everything from soap making to cooking.

Jojoba
Technically, jojoba contains more wax than oil, but is the most similar to the skin's natural oil. It is absorbed easily into the skin without clogging pores which makes it great for massages, facial care, and baths.

Avocado
Often used for dry skin and body creams. Avocado oil is known to increase the production of the skin's natural oils, so it is sometimes avoided for use in facial care.

Sweet Almond
One of the best oils for dry, sensitive skin, and is a great source of vitamin E. It has strong anti-aging, anti-inflammatory, moisturizing properties, and aids in wound healing.

Herbal Infused Oil: Slow Method

The blend below will later be used to create an array of topical products on both days 52 and 53. Be sure to choose an oil or blend of oils that are suitable for your skin type. The herbs selected are gentle on the skin and generally regarded as safe for both adults and children.

Take note of the oil as it steeps. What changes happen in the color, scent, and viscosity?

Floral Healing Oil

1/3 cup dried chamomile
1/3 cup dried lavender
1/3 cup dried rose petal
1 1/4 cup avocado, sweet almond, jojoba or blend

Combine all herbs in a sterilized mason jar, and pour oil over top. Use a clean spoon to thoroughly mix and remove all air bubbles.

Place a small piece of natural wax paper on the top of the jar (to protect the infusion from any plastic or chemical coating on the lid), and screw on lid.

Place container in a slightly warm, dark spot. Let stand for 4-6 weeks, shaking every few days to encourage mixing and to ensure herbs remain below the surface of the liquid.

Once infused, line a fine mesh sieve with cheesecloth and strain the infusion. Use the cheese cloth to squeeze out as much oil as possible.

Discard the herbs, and store the oil in a glass jar in a cool dark place. Use as desired.

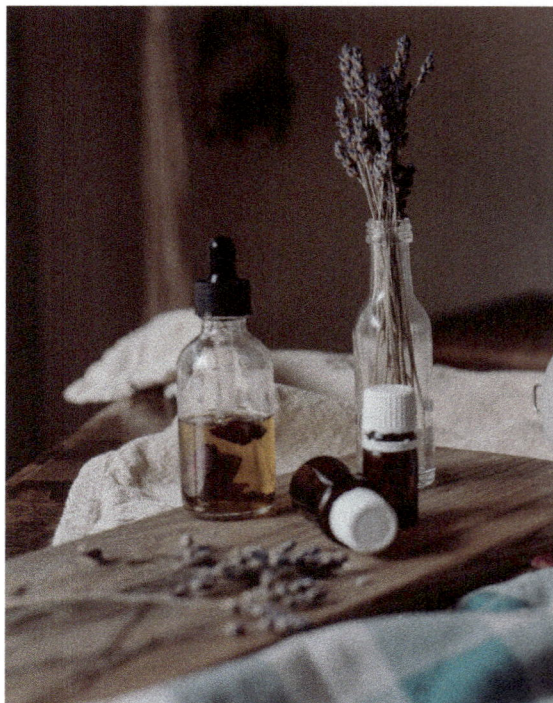

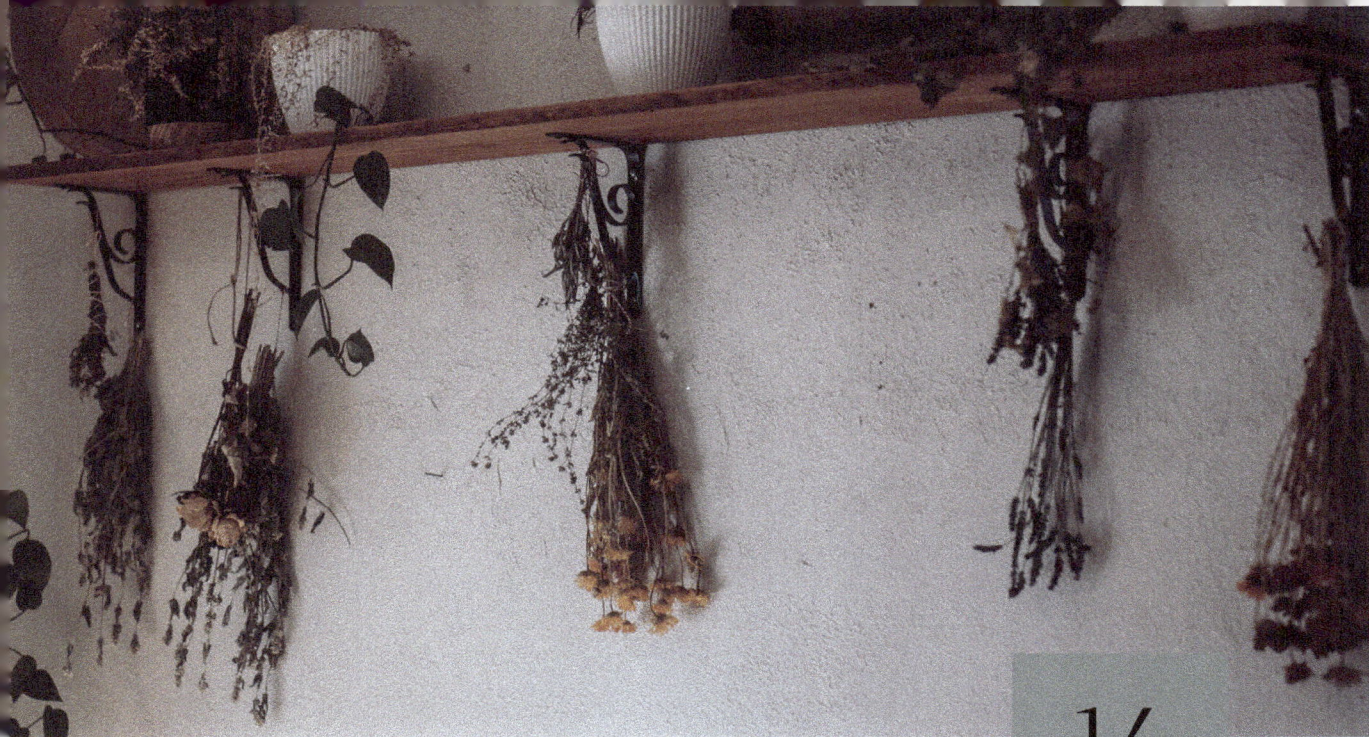

Dry Herbs 2 Ways

Learning to preserve herbs whether they are from a market, wild foraged, or home grown is an important skill. Poorly preserved herbs can lead to mold and fungal growth, which can result in sickness. Additionally, poorly preserved herbs will not be as medicinally potent as properly preserved ones.

Air Dry

This method works by allowing herbs to release their liquid into the air naturally. Air drying works best in a dry, dark environment. Stemmed herbs can be gathered into small bunches and tied together with a string or rubber band. Hang these herbs stem side up and they will dry in a few days to a couple weeks. They can be hung in cabinets, or with a paper bag over top to keep from gathering dust. Make sure that the herbs are allowed air movement to prevent from growing mold. Herbs or flowers without stems can be laid on a screen or tray in a dark, dry place.

Oven or Dehydrator Method

This method uses low heat to dry herbs at a faster rate. Place the herbs on a cookie sheet or dehydrator tray, less than one inch deep, at low heat (less than 180F) for several hours. The length of time will depend on the water content of the herb and the thickness. For example small leaves and flowers like lemon balm may dry in 1-3 hours, whereas roots may take 3-5, and lemon slices may take 6 or more.

With both methods, you will know if the herbs are dry when they become brittle and crumble easily.

15

Sweet Cinnamon Decoction

A decoction is a method of extracting the flavor and medicinal qualities of heavier, woodier plant matter – such as roots or seeds – by boiling them in water for about 20 minutes or more. The result is similar to that of an herbal tea or an infusion.

For comparison, brew a cup of tea with the same ingredients and compare it with the decoction. What are the differences in smell, color, and flavor?

Sweet Cinnamon Decoction

2 cinnamon sticks
2 tsp dandelion root
1 tsp licorice root
4 cardamom pods
3 cups cold water

Combine all ingredients in a pot. Cover and bring to a low simmer over medium heat.

Let simmer for 20-45 minutes.

Let cool and strain. Use as desired.

Note: Once the decoction is removed from heat, more delicate herbs, like leaves and flowers, can be added to steep for as long as desired prior to straining.

Sugar can be added in the last 5 minutes of simmering to create a simple syrup, like the one used in day 16. If you prefer to use honey, add it after the decoction has been removed from heat and strained.

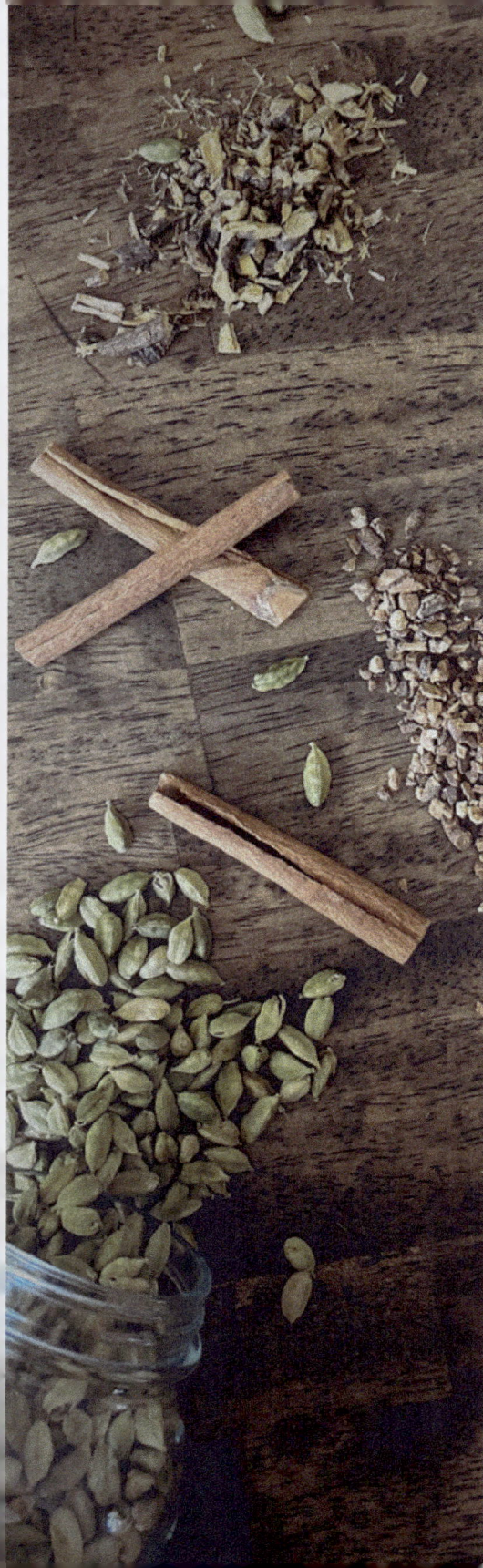

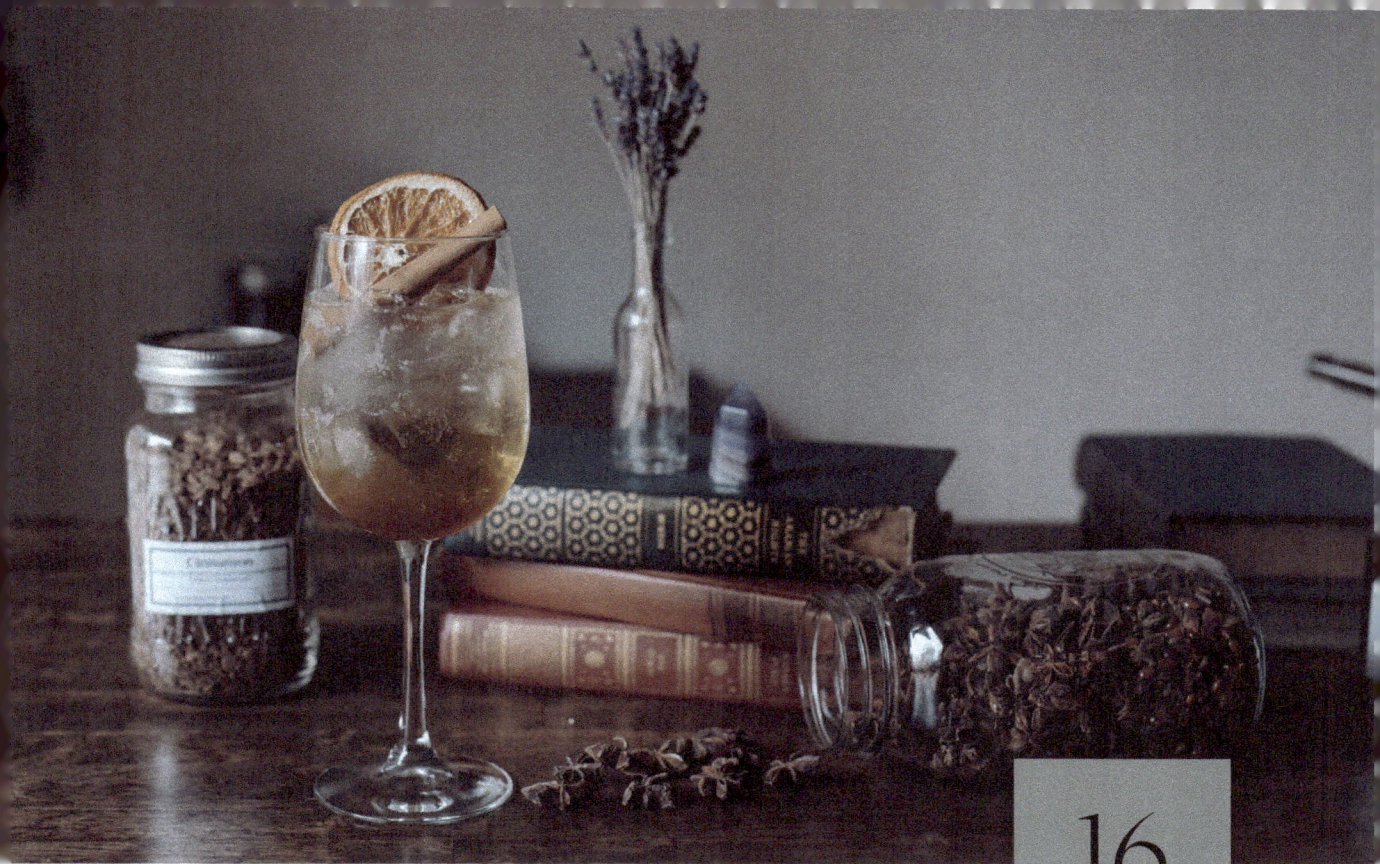

Sweet Cinnamon Herbal Soda

Herbal sodas are a great way to enjoy a refreshing drink with the additional benefit of a medicinal dose of herbs. They are often much healthier than store bought versions, typically containing colorants and preservatives. Since any herb or fruit can be made into a simple syrup, the flavor possibilities are virtually endless.

Use the sweet cinnamon decoction (from day 15) to make a simple syrup using 2-3 cups of sugar. To make the syrup, slightly warm the decoction on the stove top until the sugar dissolves, about 2-3 minutes.

Sweet Cinnamon Herbal Soda

Ice
1 oz Sweet Cinnamon Simple Syrup
6-8 oz club soda
orange slice or cherry (optional garnish)

Add ice in a glass or mason jar.

Pour in simple syrup. Top with club soda, garnish and enjoy.

Learn about Herbal Actions

Each herb is attributed with a list of actions. These actions describe how the herb affects the body. Listed below are some of the most common herbal actions, and their simplest descriptions. This is not an exhaustive list, but will give an overview of many common actions.

Adaptogen: Aids the body in adapting to stress, prevents mitochondrial dysfunction, and supports the adrenal system.

Analgesic: Soothes and relieves pain.

Anti-microbial/Antiseptic: Helps to destroy or resist microbial growth including bacteria, viruses, and fungi.

Anti-pyretic/Febrifuge: Reduces fever temperatures.

Anti-spasmodic: Reduces voluntary or involuntary muscle spasms.

Anxiolytic: Relieves mental and physical symptoms of anxiety.

Aperient: Gently stimulates the bowels.

Aphrodisiac: Stimulates sexual desire. The mechanism by which this occurs varies depending on the plant's constituents but may involve increasing blood flow to the pelvis, relaxing the nervous and musculoskeletal systems, or supplying nutrients that nourish reproductive organs.

Astringent: Contracts or tightens the tissues. Usually cooling, draining, and drying.

Bitter: Triggers bitter taste receptors, having an effect on the gastrointestinal, cardiovascular, nervous, and endocrine systems. Most notably, bitter tonics stimulate the secretion of digestive juices. Further discussion of bitters can be found on day 43.

Carminative: Reduce gas, intestinal griping, and cramping pain.

Cholagogue/Choleretic: Increases secretion of bile from the liver to aid in digestion.

Demulcent: Cooling, moistening, often mucilaginous. Heals mucous membranes by forming a protecting coating over irritated/inflamed mucosa.

Diaphoretic: Induces perspiration; often used in fever. Constitutionally drying.

Diuretic: Increases the drainage of accumulated fluid from the tissues, and/or enhances the flow of urine. Constitutionally drying.

Emmenagogue: Stimulates menstruation.

Emollient: Relaxes and soothes the skin or mucous membrane, making it soft or supple. Similar to demulcent, but is used topically and not internally.

Expectorant: Expels mucous from the respiratory tract.

Galactagogue: Stimulates the production and/or flow of milk.

Hemostatic/Styptic: Stops bleeding.

Hypertensive: Increases elevated systolic and diastolic blood pressure.

Immunomodulating: Modulates the body's immune system. Immune stimulants will stimulate the immune system to aid the body in resisting infection, often used on a short-term basis for acute infections.

Laxative: Promotes normal bowel movements. May relieve constipation through stimulation, moistening, or bulking of waste.

Lymphatic/Lymphagogue: Stimulates activity of the lymphatic system. Generally supports the lymphatic organs, and the bodies waste removal pathways.

Nervine: Acts on the nerves.

Nutritive: Rich in nutrients, these are are often eaten as foods.

Sedative: Calms and soothes the mind and body.

Stimulant: Increases energy or activity.

Tonic: Herbs that strengthen, nourish, and restore function to an organ or system. Usually organ or system-specific, but can act on the whole body.

Trophorestorative: Nourishes/restores the function of an organ or system.

Vulnerary: Aids in wound healing.

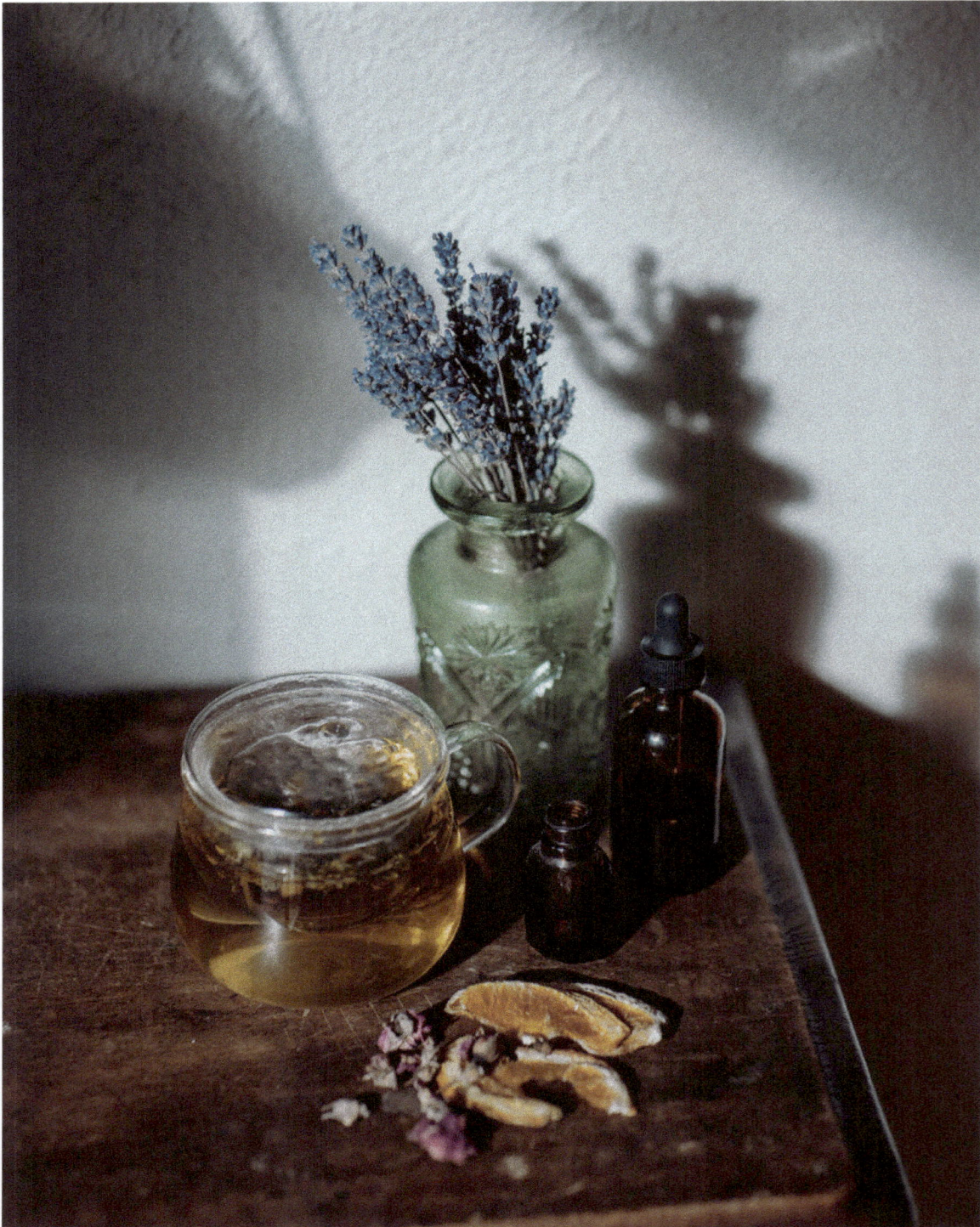

Herbal Actions Activity

FIll in the boxes with herbs that have the corresponding action listed on top. Some of these herbs will be referenced throughout the book. However, reviewing a book from the additional sources on day 100 can be helpful.

Bitter	Anitseptic	Expectorant
	Thyme	*Thyme*

Vulnerary	Adaptogen	Diuretic

Nervine	Carminative	Demulcent
	Thyme	

19

Nourishing Herbal Infusions

A nourishing herbal infusion is a long steeped tea using nutritive herbs. The benefit to a longer steeping time is that it allows water to be absorbed into the plant matter, breaking it down on a cellular level. This allows larger quantities of vitamins and minerals to be released, creating a truly power-packed drink. It's a great way to increase your daily intake of vitamins and minerals, especially for those with compromised digestion.

Herbs to use: nettles, oat straw, red clover, chickweed, hawthorne, violet, burdock, dandelion leaf, mullein, plantain, or linden.

Tips:
- Use dried herbs. Minerals and other phytochemicals found in nutritive herbs are made more accessible by drying.
- Avoid aromatic herbs, as they can be overwhelming and are typically not nutritive.
- If the infusion becomes too bitter for your taste, sweeten with honey, or mix with juice or an aromatic tea (like peppermint) that's been made separately.

Suggestion: use nettle for this recipe and compare it to the tea prepared on day 20.

Nourishing Herbal Infusion Recipe
1 oz dried nettle
1 qt hot water

Weigh out herbs in a quart sized jar. Fill jar with boiling water, and let stand until it reaches room temperature. Transfer to fridge, and continue steeping for 4-24 hours.

Strain and use as desired.

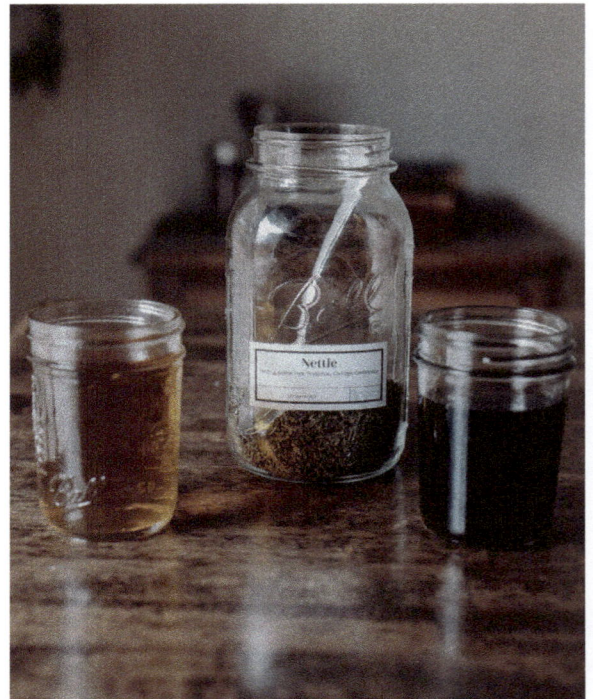

20

Make a Cup of Nettle Tea

Nettle (Urtica dioica) is a highly nutritive herb that is great for maintaining health, when drank regularly. It is astringent, tonic, diuretic, antihistamine, and anti-inflammatory, in addition to other actions.

Make a cup of nettle tea using 1-2 tsp for every 8 oz of water. Compare the flavor of the hot tea, to the cold nourishing herbal infusion made on day 19.

Record your thoughts here:

Go for a Plant Walk

Plant walks are a great way to learn about plants and plant families. Take a stroll anywhere that there are plants and try to identify as many as you can. See how many medicinal plants, toxic plants, and ornamental plants you can identify. Below are a list of some common wild medicinal herbs:

Broadleaf Plantain (Plantago major) A plant with a long history of use for everything from bowel issues to wound-healing. It is anti-microbial, anti-inflammatory, and astringent; helping to heal and draw out impurities of the skin. It can be found growing in poor soils, lawns, and in cracks of concrete.

Chickweed (Stellaria media) Best when picked in early spring, chickweed is famous for its high nutrient content, as well as reducing inflammation, supporting immune health, and fighting obesity. It is often used in spring tonic recipes, helping to move lymph fluid in the body. It can be used dried, or tossed fresh into salads or green pestos, like the one shown on day 25.

Violet (Viola spp.) Another early spring favorite that is highly nutritive as well as beneficial to both the respiratory and lymphatic systems. Every part of the violet is edible, from the root to the flower. When used as a tea or simple syrup, the flowers create a purple or pink concoction – adding a bit of fun to your typical drinks.

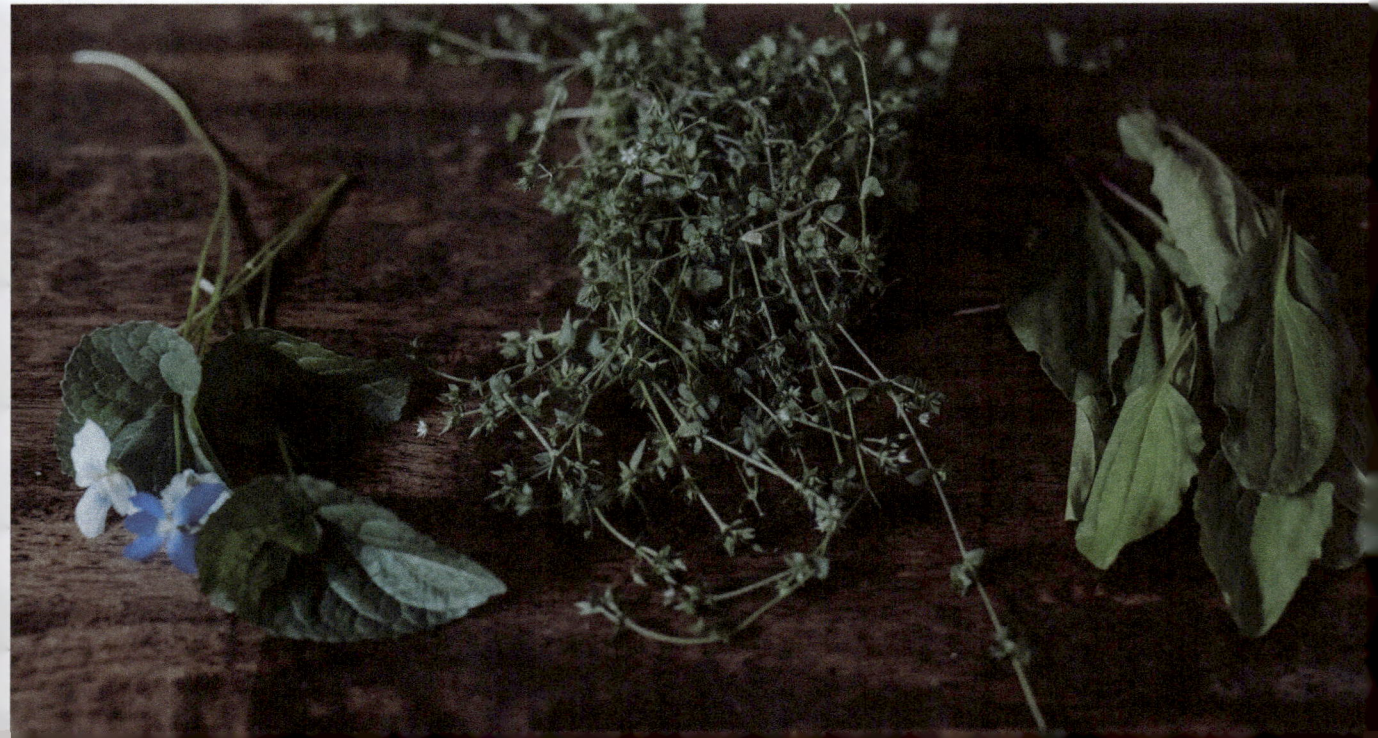

Take a moment to write down the plants that you were able to identify as well as the date, location, temperature, and any other notes you may find important:

Make a Poultice

A poultice is a soft, moist mass of plant material that is applied to the body and kept in place with a cloth. They can be used to relieve soreness, inflammation, and promote wound healing – such as in the case of infection, sprain, or bruising. A poultice can be utilized to help remove cysts, or help with pain associated with arthritis.

Plantain (Plantago major) is probably the most common herbal poultice, since it is readily available and often used for common issues like bug bites, bee stings, and minor burns and cuts. Plantain is anti-inflammatory, vulnerary, astringent, and antiseptic. These actions together make a wonderful healing helper.

The simplest version of this type of poultice is made by chewing a freshly picked leaf and placing it on the affected area, such as a bug bite or bee sting. The recipe below, however, is for a larger poultice that does not include spit.

Poultice Instructions

1 cup fresh herbs; such as plantain, chickweed, dandelion leaf, comfrey, ginger, garlic, calendula, lavender, or yarrow

Roughly chop the herbs into manageable pieces, about 1/2 inch square. Transfer to a mortar and pestle.

Use the mortar and pestle to crush herbs until they become a pulpy mass.

Spread crushed herbs onto the desired area, and wrap with a layer of gauze or muslin to hold the paste in place. You may even wish to apply a layer of plastic wrap to the outside of the finished poultice, which will help keep it in place and reduce mess.

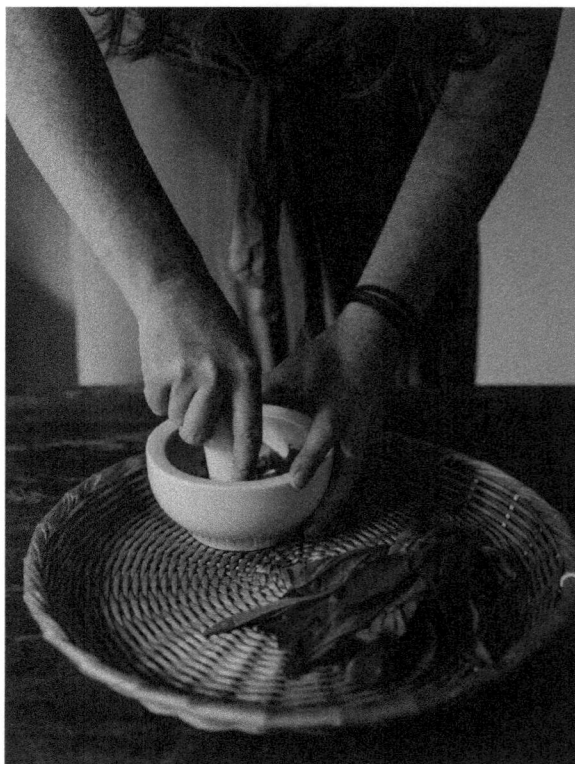

Calendula Infused Oil: Heat Method

Herbal oils can be made several ways. On day 13, a preparation of herbal infused oils were made using the slow extraction method. This recipe utilizes a heat extraction method, requiring much less time while still producing a potent product. This is a preferred method when fresh plant matter is being used to avoid potential mold and spoilage.

Calendula (Calendula officinalis) is a powerful healing plant that has been used topically for centuries for healing minor wounds, bites, stings, rashes, and the like. Not only does it help with tissue healing, but the pain and inflammation associated with it as well. In salve form, calendula can help with small cuts, rashes, dermatitis, skin lightening, and repairing sun damage.

Calendula Infused Oil

1/2 cup calendula flowers
1/2 cup olive, or avocado oil

Place herbs and oil in a mason jar, or the bowl of a double boiler. Make sure herbs remain below the level of the oil, adding more as needed.

Place jar of herbs in a Crockpot or stock pot with water, keeping the jar lifted off the bottom of the pot with a canning tray or the like.

Gently heat herbs over very low heat (90° and 120° F) for 3-5 hours.

Remove from heat, and allow to cool before straining.

Use this oil to make the salve described on day 24.

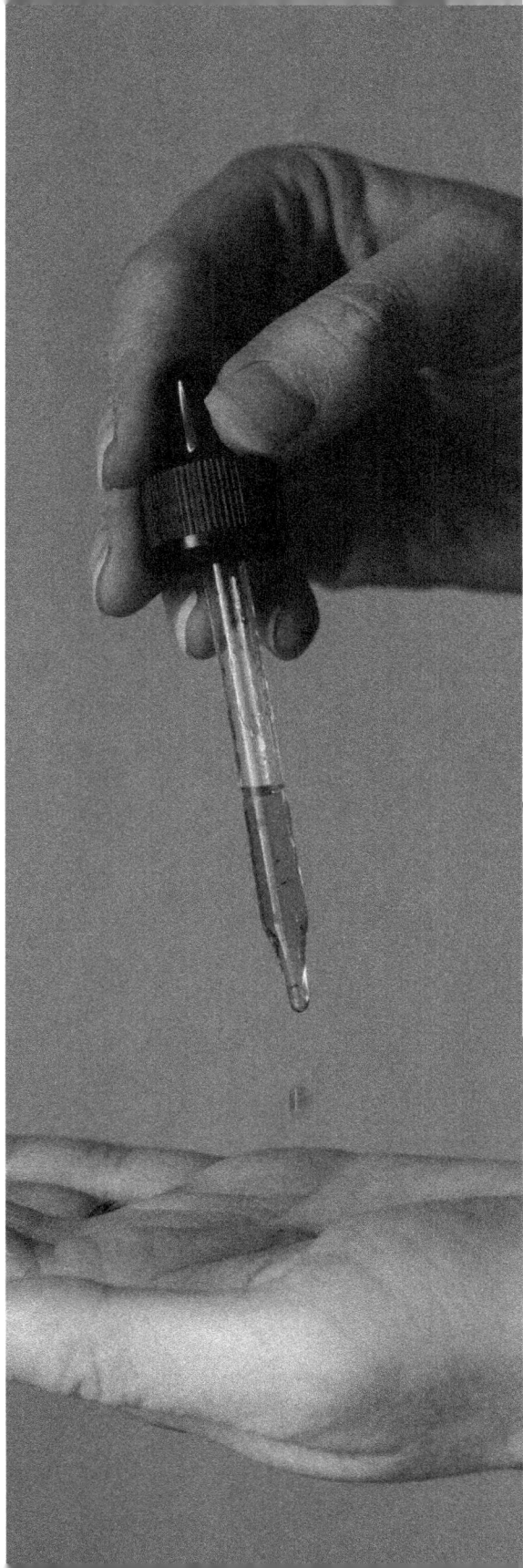

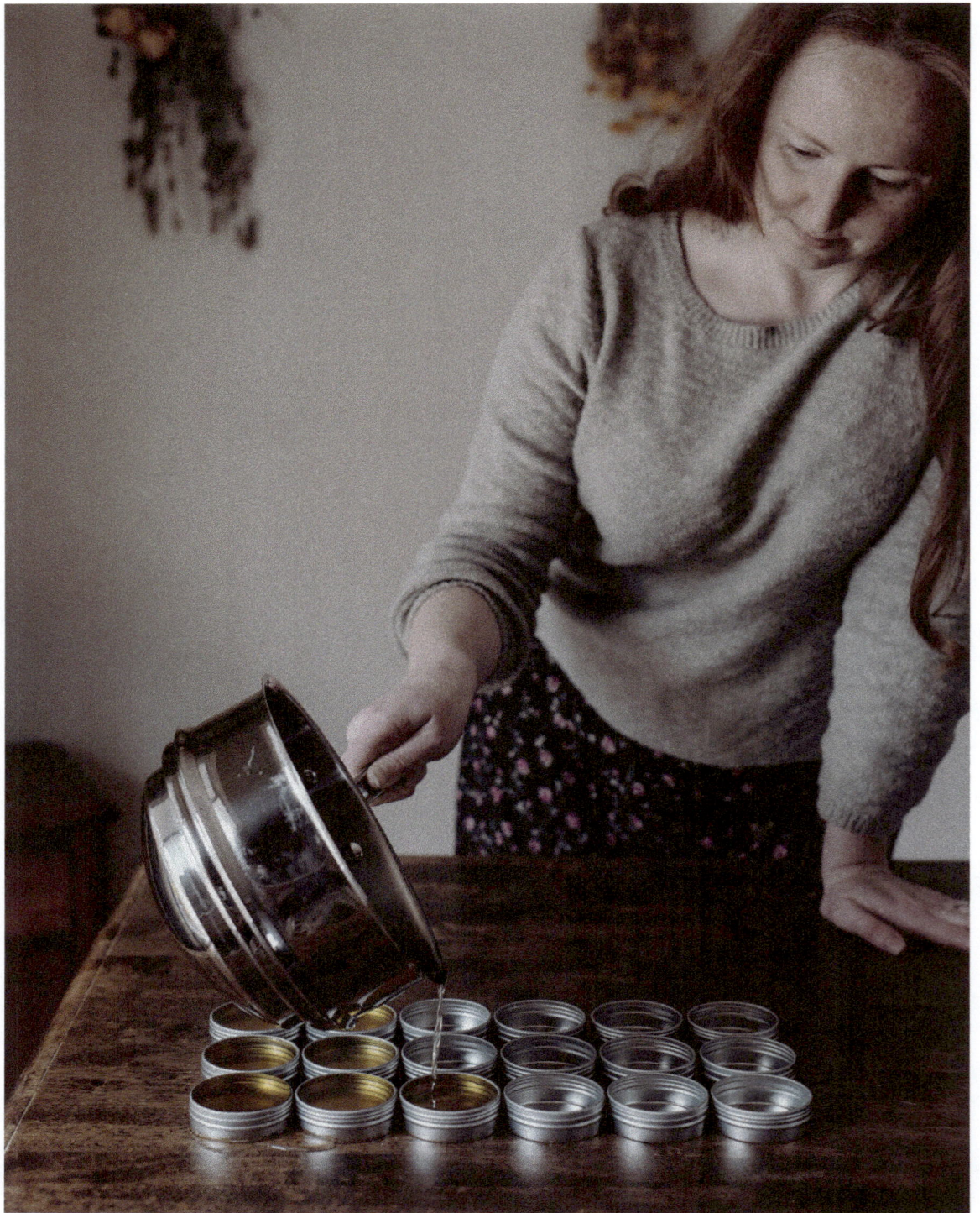

Calendula Salve

Salves and balms are ointments that are solid at room temperature and are used to administer herbal-infused oil to the skin. They are typically made by melting together infused oils with wax and other ingredients such as vitamin E, essential oils, or butters (such as shea or cocoa).

Salves and balms can be used in a similar fashion as lotions to help heal cracked, dry, or damaged skin and to ease the pain of bug bites, stings, and small abrasions. They are a great option for rashes and for easing the symptoms of dermatitis. Additionally, salves made with strong smelling herbs can be used as solid perfumes, or even tinted with mica or plant powders to be used as makeup.

Once made, salves have a shelf life of anywhere from 6 months to 3 years depending on the oil used. It's always a good idea to check the shelf life of the oil you are using, especially when making long-lasting salves.

Salve Instructions

1 cup calendula infused oil (day 23)
1/4 cup beeswax
2 drops vitamin E
20-30 drops Essential Oils (optional)

Combine calendula oil and wax in the top of a double boiler. Fill bottom of the double boiler with 2-3 inches of water ,and bring to a light simmer to gently heat the oil and wax.

Continue to heat while stirring occasionally, until all wax has dissolved. Be sure to heat until there are no ripples in the surface of the oil, this means that the wax is fully dissolved.

Remove from heat, and stir in the vitamin E and essential oils.

Carefully pour mixture into sealable jars or tins to cool. Once cooled, the salve should be solid.

To use: Rub fingers across the surface of the salve to pick up a small amount and apply to the affected area as desired.

Note: Avoid "hot" or citrus essential oils when using topically or for damaged skin. Good oils for this recipe are lavender, chamomile, jasmine, or rose.

25

Mixed Greens Pesto

Pesto is a traditional sauce made from a mixture of herbs and oil that is pounded or crushed together into a smooth paste. Most of us know pesto as an Italian condiment that utilizes basil, garlic, pine nuts and olive oil. However, it can be made with a wide array of herbs. This particular recipe is more basic, utilizing walnuts; as they are more easily accessible and lend a light flavor to various greens. It can be used as a topping for sandwiches, as a dip, a spread for crackers, or as a sauce for pasta or rice.

Other fresh herbs to use in pesto include: dandelion leaf, chickweed, basil, tulsi (holy basil), oregano, lemon balm, ramp greens, wild mustard, wood sorrel, violet leaf, dead nettle, plantain, lambs quarter, wild lettuces, and more. Each herb lends its own flavor to the sauce; feel free to experiment with the proportions to create a flavor that you enjoy!

Basic Pesto Recipe

1/2 cup walnuts, cashews, or pine nuts
2-3 cloves garlic, minced
1/2 tsp salt
1/4 tsp freshly ground black pepper
3 cups loosely packed green herbs, lightly chopped
1 Tbsp lemon juice
1/2 cup extra virgin olive oil
1/4 cup freshly grated Parmesan cheese (or nutritional
yeast, to taste)

Classic preparation: In the bowl of a mortar and pestle, crush walnuts until they become a paste. Add garlic, salt, and pepper, and continue to crush into a well blended paste. Blend in greens, lemon juice, and oil until well blended. Stir in Parmesan cheese to finish, and serve.

Food Processor version: In the bowl of a food processor, combine walnuts, garlic, salt and pepper. Lightly pulse to blend. Add greens, lemon juice, olive oil, and Parmesan, pulsing until a smooth paste forms. Add more olive oil if needed to create the desired consistency.

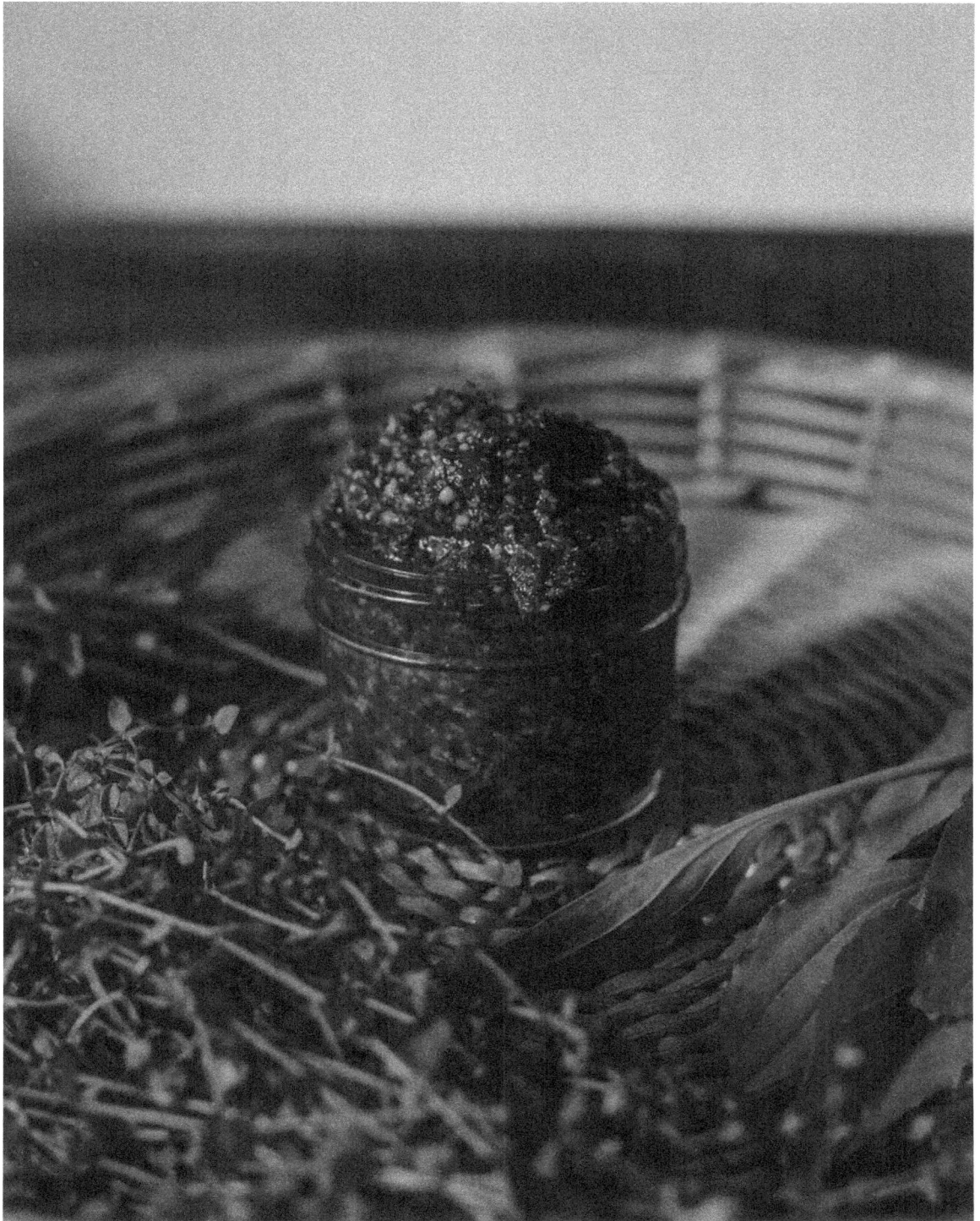

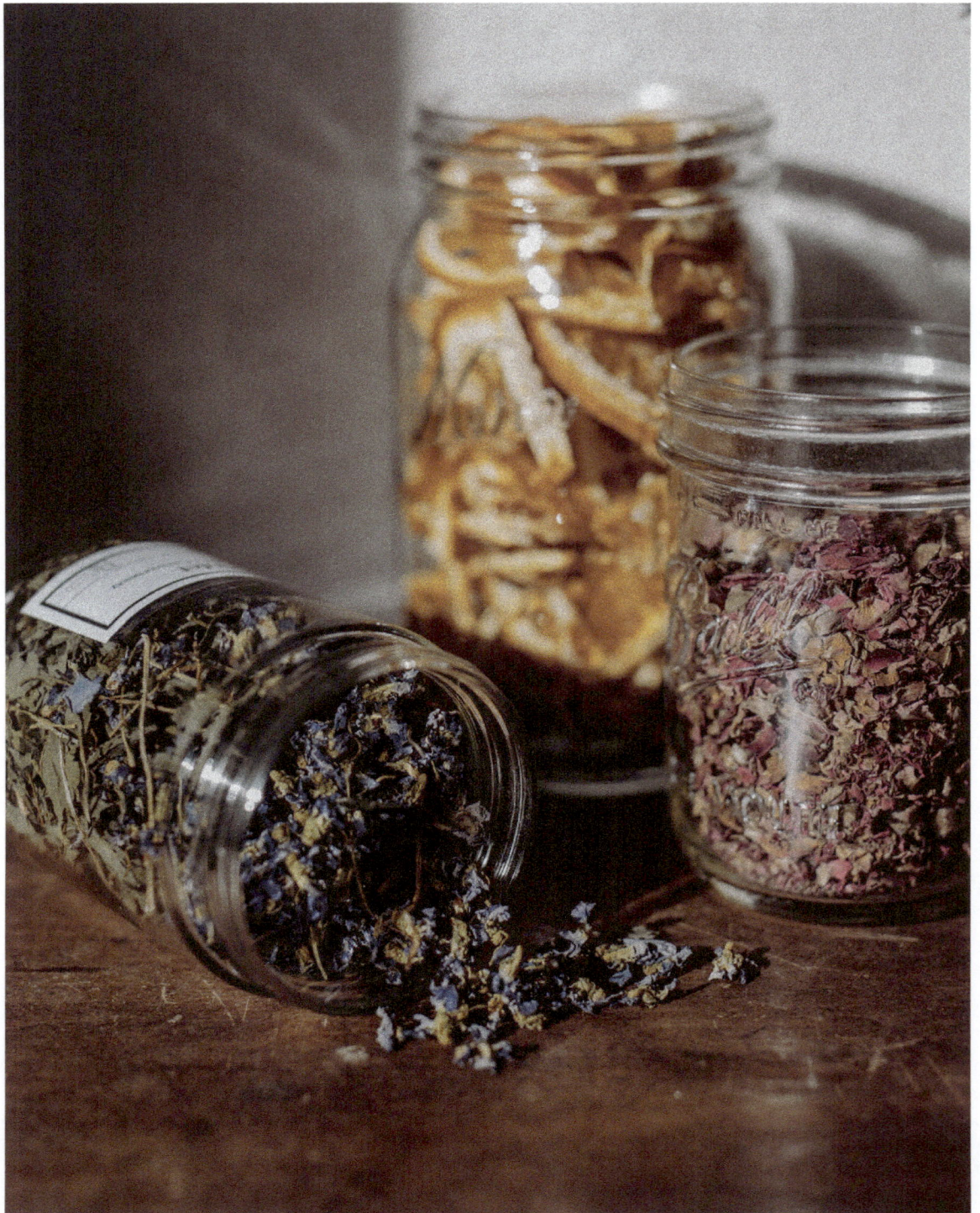

Learn about Herbs for Skincare

Calendula (Calendula officinalis) - With anti-inflammatory and skin-healing properties, Calendula has become one of the most famous skincare and wound healing herbs. It is beneficial for all skin types, but especially for acne-prone or sensitive skin.

Chamomile (Matricaria chamomilla)- A calming herb for both mind and body, chamomile is a great choice for red and irritated skin. Its emollient properties make it another great choice for sensitive, dry, or acne-prone skin.

Rose Petals (Rosa spp.) - A beloved beauty herb that brings moisture, nourishment, and anti-aging properties that can even skin tone and smooth out fine lines and wrinkles for all skin types.

Lavender (Lavendula spp.) - Another herb that can balance and nourish all skin types, but is great for balancing the skin's natural oil production and stimulating new cell growth, providing a youthful glow.

Hibiscus (Hibiscus sabdariffa)- High in antioxidants and vitamins; hibiscus is known for it's ability to help repair damaged skin, for evening skin texture and elasticity, smoothing out wrinkles, and balance complexion. It is best for mature, dry, or sun-damaged skin.

Plantain (Plantago major) - Often used for it's wound-healing properties, plantain can also help to pull out impurities, smooth out scars, reduce inflammation and acne, as well as balance the skin's microbiome.

Rosemary (Rosemarinus officinalis) - Known to improve blood flow, rosemary is great for improving dull and mature skin, repairing sun damage, reducing inflammation and puffiness, as well as improving fine lines and wrinkles.

Nettle (Urtica dioica) - The astringent properties of nettle make it great for tightening and toning the skin. It's beneficial for reducing redness, balancing sebum production, and supporting skin elasticity.

Peppermint (Mentha x piperita) - Cooling and soothing to the skin, mint is also known to help cleanse, reduce puffiness, and to even skin tone.

Tulsi/Holy Basil (Ocimum tenuiflorum) - Often used in toners to rebalance the skin, promote skin-brightening, and to prevent or reduce hyper-pigmentation. Anti-bacterial, anti-inflammatory, stress reducing.

Herbal Clay Mask

1 Tbsp powdered herb blend of choice (see Day 26 for herbal suggestions)
2 Tbsp bentonite or similar clay
1 1/2 Tbsp water or apple cider vinegar

Sift together herb blend and clay.

Stir in water or apple cider vinegar to create a paste.

To use: Spread paste across the skin with fingers or a gentle brush. Let stand for 5-15 minutes, depending on skin type (read instructions on the chosen clay before use). Rinse off with warm water.

Those with sensitive skin should complete a 1-2 inch test patch on the inner arm before use.

Note: To powder your own herbs, combine them in a clean coffee grinder. Once they are mostly powdered, sift them through a fine sieve to remove any large pieces that could abrade the skin.

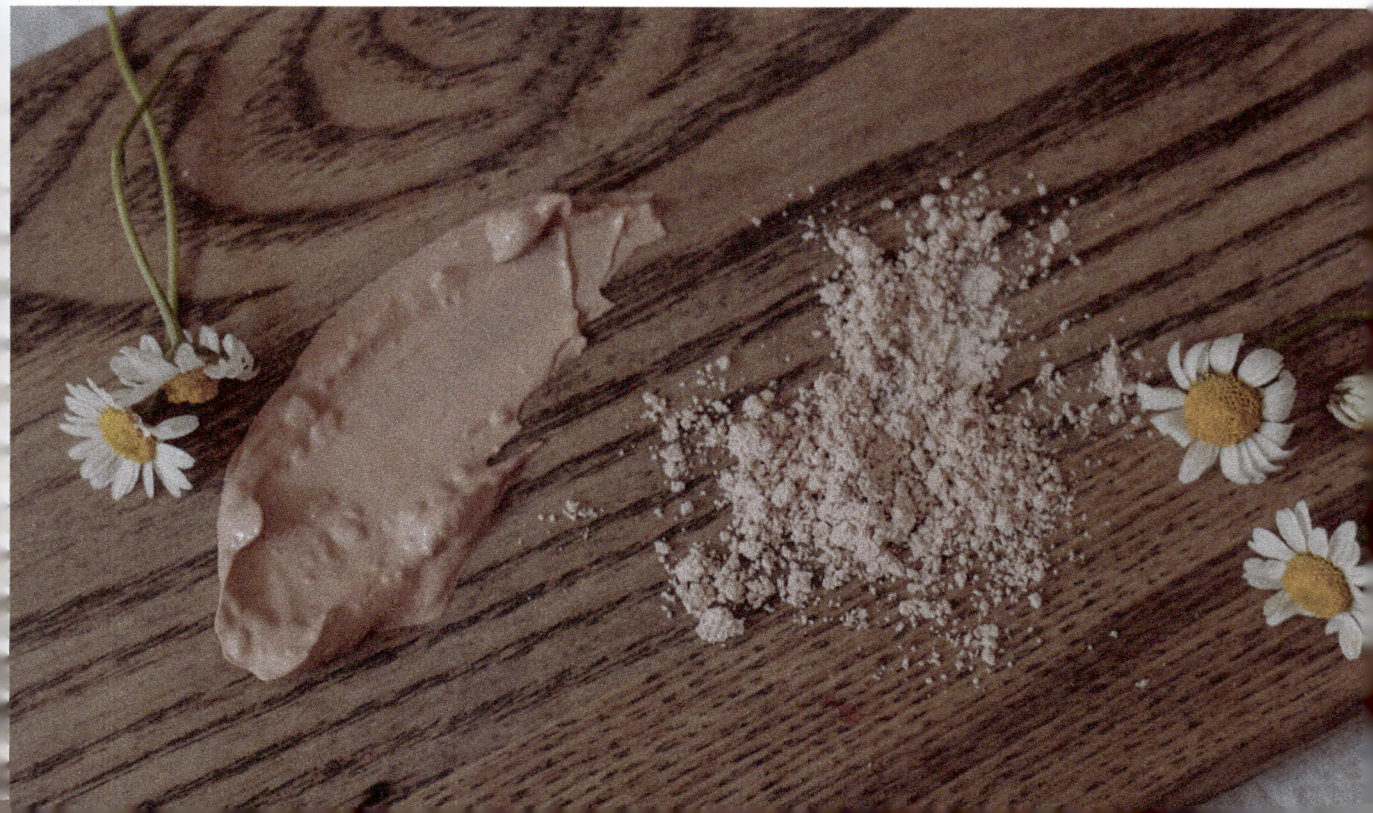

4 Thieves Vinegar

The legend of The Four Thieves has many variations, with the most common story revolving around four people who lived through the plague of Marseilles, France in the 1700s. They were arrested for robbing the homes and corpses of the deceased. Once arrested, the thieves were questioned on how they remained healthy, despite constant exposure to the illness, sparking the trade of their secret blend of herbs in order to spare their lives.

Over the years, many variations of this recipe have appeared with numerous claims and uses. In modern times, studies have shown the efficacy of these herbs and their power to fight viruses, fungus, bacteria, and more.

Use this recipe for everything from a delicious salad dressing or marinade, to house cleaning and pest control. Flip to Day 56 for specific recipes and uses.

4 Thieves Vinegar

1 Tbsp dried sage
1 tsp dried lavender
1 tsp dried rosemary
1/2 tsp dried thyme
1/2 tsp black peppercorns
1/2 tsp cloves
16 oz raw apple cider vinegar

Place herbs in a pint jar and fill with lukewarm apple cider vinegar.

Place a small piece of natural wax paper on the top of the jar (to protect the infusion as discussed on day 07), and screw on the lid.

Allow to extract for four weeks, shaking regularly.

Strain vinegar into a sealable glass jar.

Store in a cool, dark place and use as desired.

If mold develops on the surface, discard.

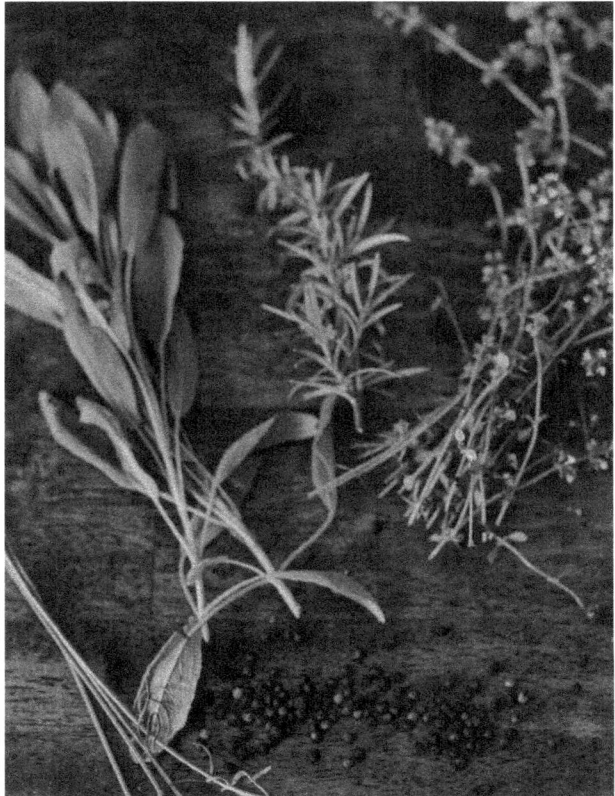

Adaptogen Hot Cocoa

Cocoa is known for being both rich and sweet, making it a great companion to the more earthy and pungent roots and mushrooms that are characteristic of many adaptogens.

Adaptogens are a class of herbs that are thought to help the body adapt to stress, by bringing the body into balance, supporting the adrenal system, and providing nutrients that help to normalize bodily processes.

This recipe is meant to be an outline. Feel free to experiment with different types of milk and adaptogen powders. Some other adaptogens to try include shatavari root, astragulus root, schisandra berries, ginseng, and epimedium.

Both reishi and maca are herbs that have gained popularity in the last few years for their powerful abilities to help the body. Reishi (Ganoderma lingzhi) especially, has been touted as an energy and brain-booster, as well as being immune-supportive. Maca (Lepidium meyenii) has been used to support elevated mood, stress management, boost libido, and support women with perimenouse symptoms.

Adaptogen Hot Cocoa

2 1/2 cups milk of choice
2 Tbsp cacao powder
1/2 tsp cinnamon
3-4 Tbsp maple syrup
pinch sea salt
1 tsp vanilla
1 tsp reishi powder
1 tsp ashwagandha powder
1 Tbsp maca powder

Combine all ingredients in a small pan and whisk until well combined. Transfer to the stove, stirring frequently over medium heat until cocoa reaches desired temperature.

Serve warm.

Makes 2 servings.

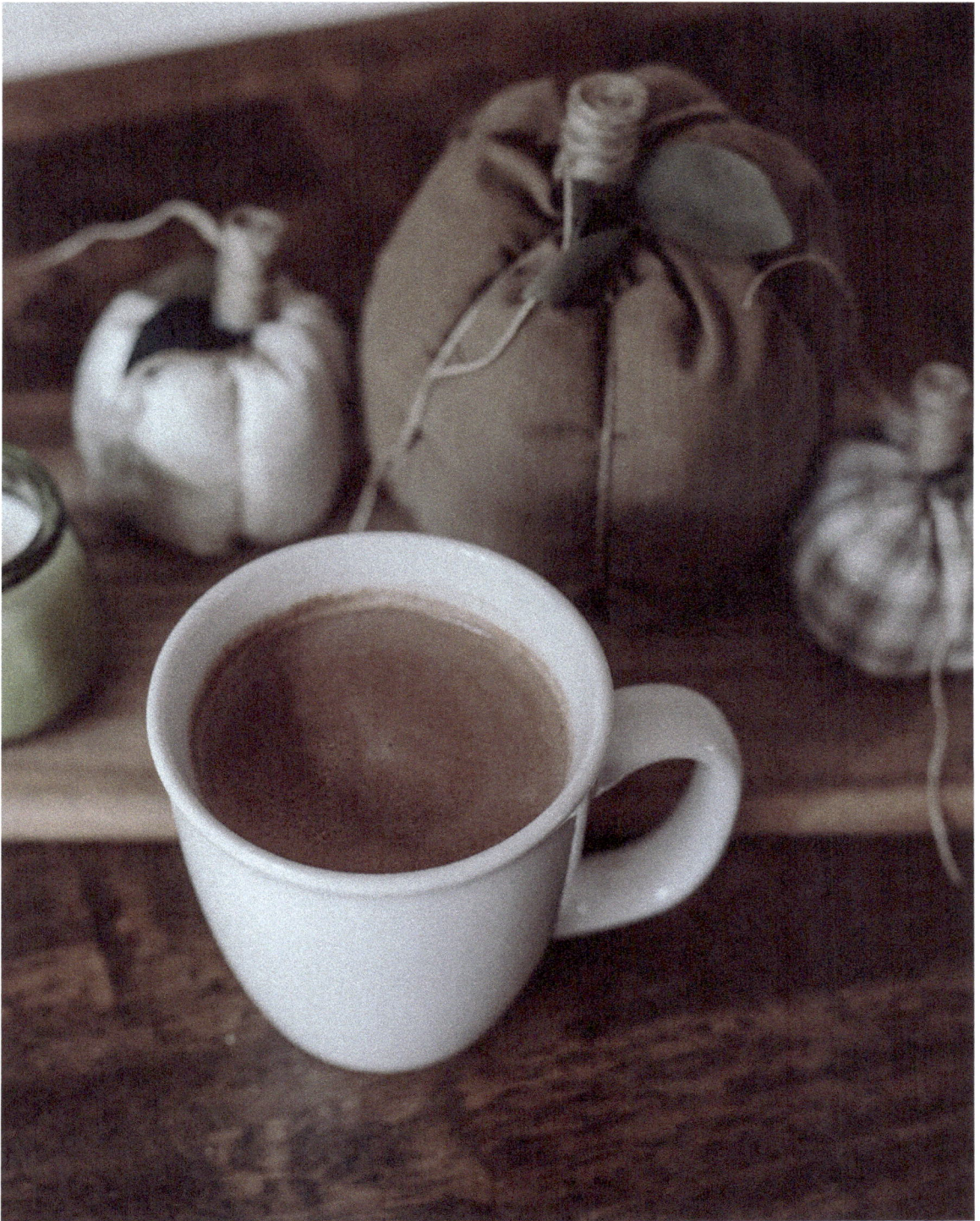

Chamomile Body Scrub

Epsom salt scrubs are a great way to help relax sore muscles, exfoliate the skin, and detox the body. Adding herbs allows the skin to absorb it's benefits, boosting the scrub's power and further helping to nourish the body.

Chamomile is an anti-inflammatory, anti-spasmodic, and calming nervine, giving it the unique ability to help ease both physical and mental stress. Adding orange in this recipe gives it a bright scent that helps to lift spirits.

Chamomile Body Scrub

1 cup fine Epsom salt
3 Tbsp powdered chamomile
1 Tbsp powdered orange peel
1/4 cup avocado or coconut oil

Combine all ingredients in a large bowl, stirring until well combined. Store in an airtight jar.

Use a handful of scrub to gently rub onto skin for 2-5 minutes, but for no longer than 10 minutes. Rinse area until clear of all salt residue. Repeat 2-3 times per week as desired.

Make an Herbal Compress

Herbal compresses are a quick and easy way to utilize herbs topically. The most basic of which require a cloth dipped into a strongly brewed herbal infusion.

For this preparation, brew a strong cup of chamomile tea and use it to dampen a cloth. There are generally two ways to prepare a stronger cup of tea. The first is to increase the amount of herbs used, from 1-2 tsps to 2-3 tsps per cup. Alternatively, you could increase the length of time steeped upwards of 10-20 minutes.

Once prepared, make sure the tea has cooled enough to avoid burning the skin. Place the cloth on the skin and let it sit for 5-10 minutes. Notice how your skin feels before and after. While using the cloth, be sure to inhale the relaxing aroma. Take a moment to relax into the preparation.

Chamomile (Matricaria chamomilla) is a great herb for topical use and has been used for centuries for skin irritations, sunburn, rashes, and sores. It has benefits for eye strain, headaches, and facial care. Chamomile is anti-inflammatory, antiseptic, and promotes wound healing. While being a powerful ally, it is gentle enough to be used with children both topically and internally from rashes (externally) to colic (used internally as a tea).

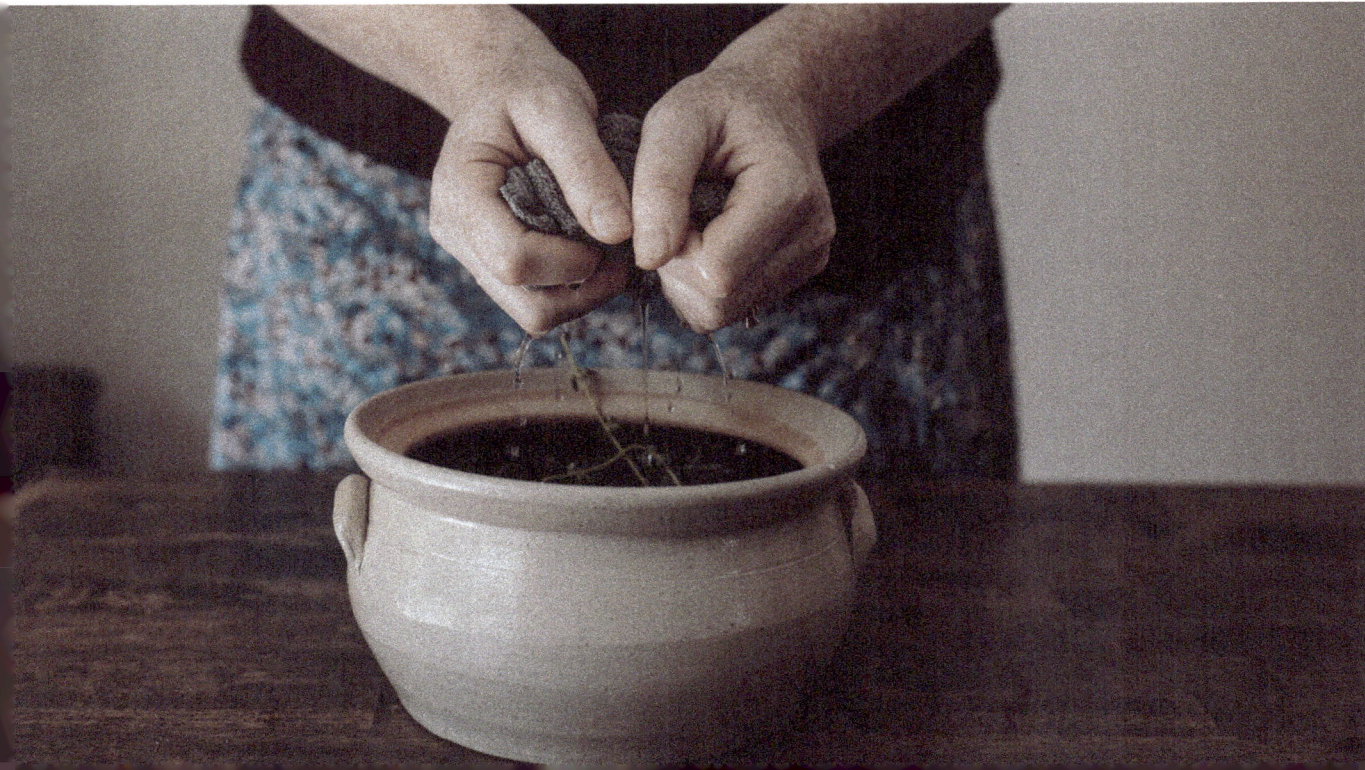

Make a Simple Tincture

A tincture is an extract of plant or animal material dissolved in alcohol. While often used in culinarily for flavor, herbal extracts can also be a powerful medicine. Tinctures are a great way to preserve plant matter for longer periods of time. Also enabling the preservation of some herbs while they are in season and at peak freshness for use at any time of year.

Tinctures are typically much stronger than teas, and therefore only require small amounts for each dose. This makes them easy to administer, especially for herbs that are not as palatable and for those who dislike tea. The adult dosage for most tinctures is usually 1-3 ml, or the amount that can fit into a single dropper. It is important to respect the recommended dose for each herb in a tincture, as overuse can result in adverse effects.

For this recipe, Ashwagandha (Withania somnifera) was chosen, for it is a powerful herb that is often touted for its adaptogenic and restorative nature. It is often employed in cases of chronic fatigue and stress. Adding this tincture to a daily mocktail, or a morning shot of water, is a great way to help support the body through stressful times. It is important to note that not every herb is beneficial for every person. It is suggested to study each herb before using medicinally on a regular basis. For those that are averse to using alcohol, you can make a glycerite, like on day 6 or a vinegar extract shown on day 11 or 28.

Additional notes:

It is important to match the alcohol strength for the herb being utilized as discussed on day 07. Also, when blending multiple herbs in a tincture, it is beneficial to tincture each herb separately, according to the preferred strength and ratio, then blend the final tinctures together.

Ashwagandha Tincture

1 oz dried ashwagandha root (by weight)
5 oz of 140 proof (70%) or higher alcohol (by volume)

Combine herb and alcohol in a sterile mason jar. If the alcohol does not cover the herb, you will need to add more. Be sure to measure the additional amount. On a label, write all ingredient measurements, and the date.

Secure the mixture with a paper lined lid. Place jar in a dark cabinet and allow the mixture to infuse for 6-8 weeks, shaking occasionally.

Turn to day 78 for more information on straining, dosage, and use.

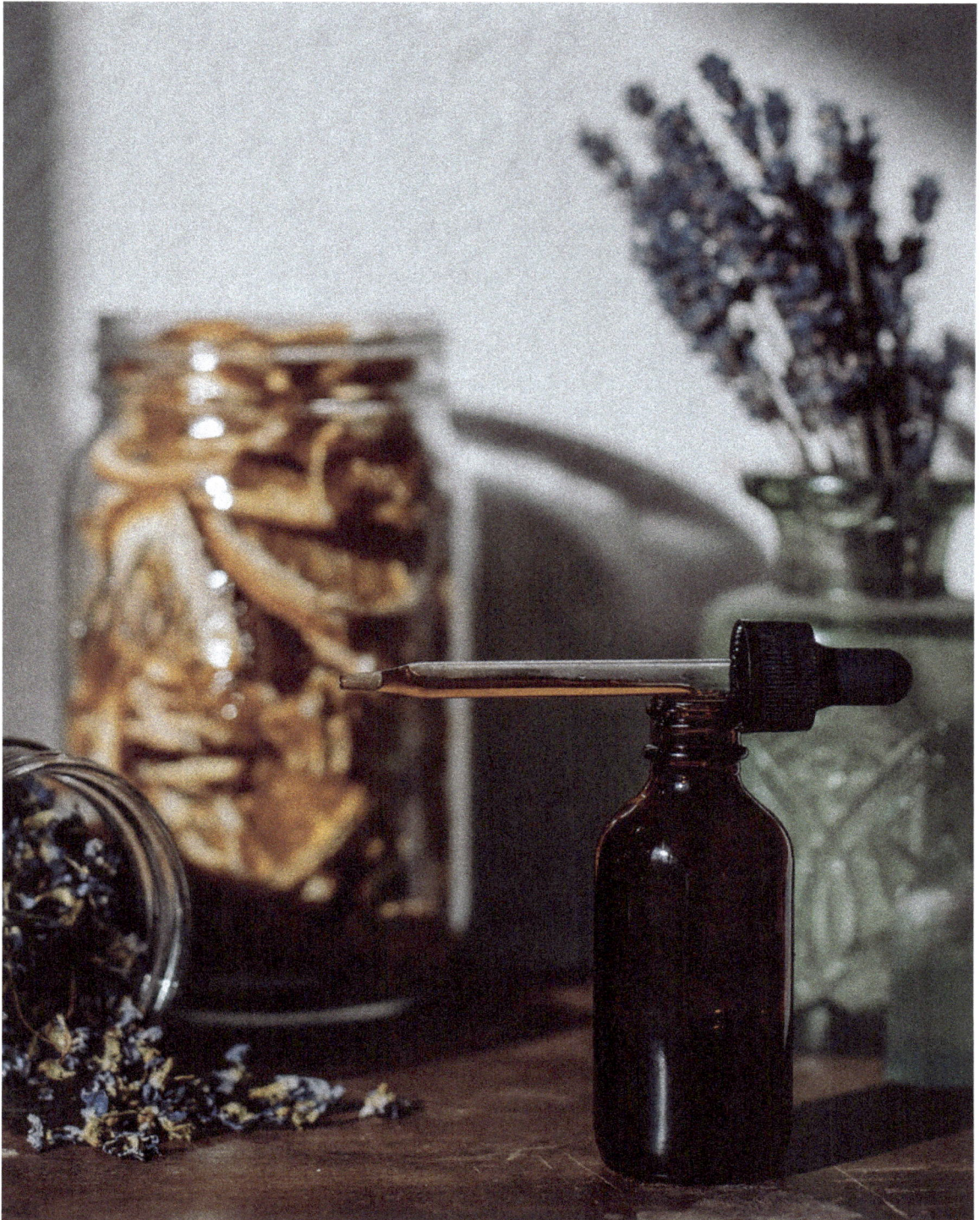

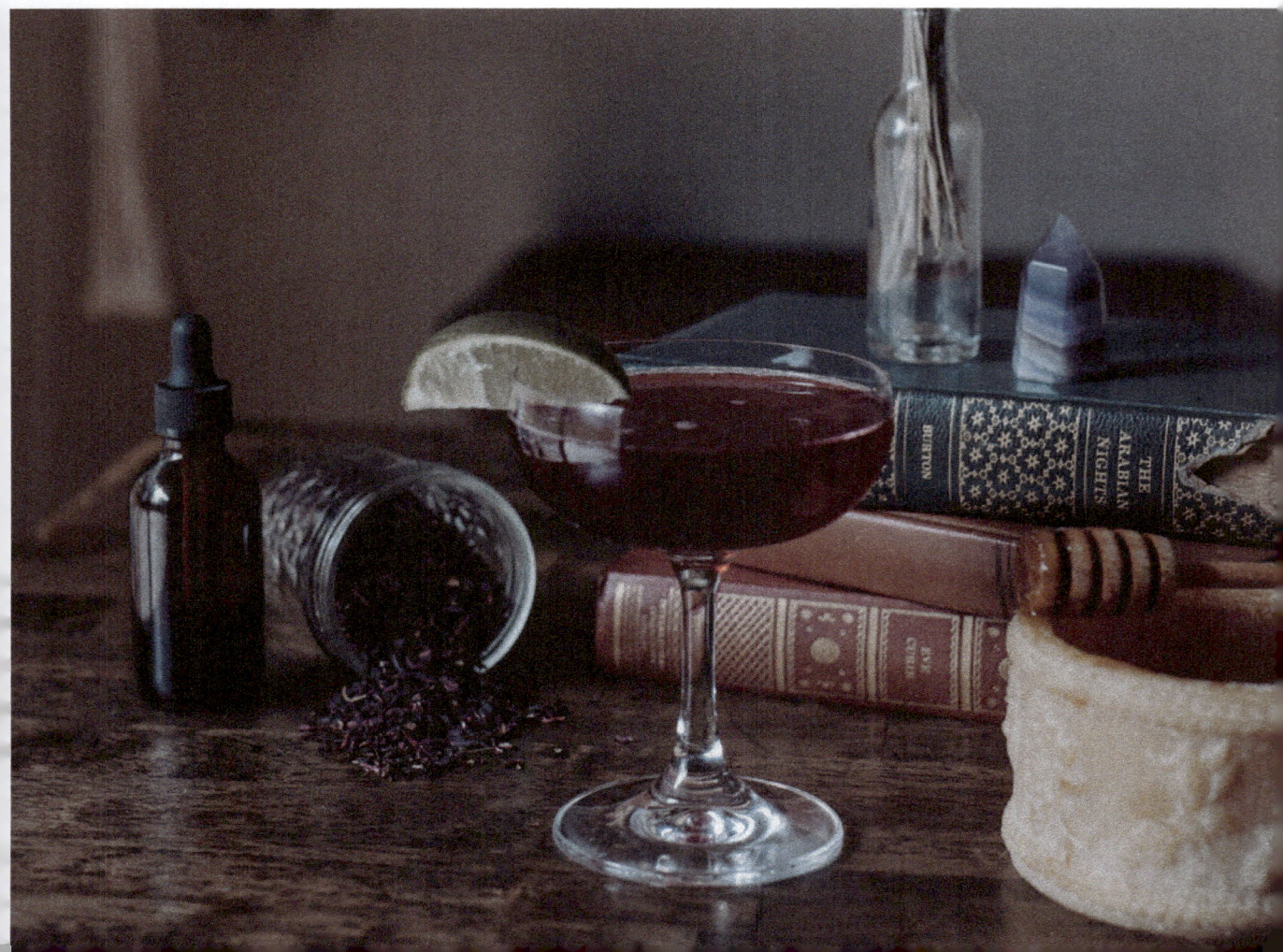

33

Decant Tulsi Hibiscus Oxymel

After 4 weeks of steeping, the Tulsi Hibiscus Oxymel made on day 11 can be strained. Use a fine mesh strainer lined with cheese cloth to separate the liquid from the plant matter. Use your hands to squeeze out as much of the liquid from the cloth as possible. Store in a sealed container in the fridge for up to 6 months.

Oxymels, like most other vinegar infusions, have many uses. They can be made into refreshing, medicinal drinks, marinades, or even salad dressings. To create a drink, simply add 1-2 oz of oxymel to seltzer or water; garnish as desired.

Blending Herbal Teas

Blending your own herbal teas can be a satisfying and useful skill, allowing you to create pleasurable teas that suit your personal needs. The three step system described here is a simple way to begin blending teas for multiple purposes.

Choose A Base

Typically, the base of the tea is the key ingredient. Whether the base is simply for flavor, or for medicinal qualities, is up to the blender. When using an herb for its medicinal qualities, it is important to keep in mind the herbal actions, energetics, and the nature of the ailment to the person who will be consuming the blend.

For example, if you are making a blend to support someone through grief, you will want to start with a base that not only supports the emotions of the person, but also their taste preferences. Do they prefer warming teas? Perhaps Tusli would be a good base. If they prefer a cooling tea, try linden or rose.

Supporting Herbs

These are selected to add flavor, or to add a complimentary affect or flavor to the base herbs. Typically, if you are using 3 parts of a base ingredient, the supporting herbs will make up 1-2 parts of the formula.

To continue our example, a tea with a base of tulsi would blend nicely with an herb like mimosa, an herb that supports grief, and is neutral in its energetics (i.e. it is not warming or cooling). This would look like 3 Tbsp tulsi and 1-2 Tbsp mimosa.

Accent Herbs

Accent herbs are the final touch to a blend, and can add a pop of flavor or help to round it out. These are usually added in smaller portions of 1/4 to 1 part.

A blend that uses tulsi and mimosa, would go well with a touch of cardamom and rose,or cinnamon, depending on personal flavor preference. Other flavorful herbs such as hibiscus, lavender, or mint will work as well.

To continue the example, you could add 1 Tbsp (1 part) cardamom pods and 2 tsp (0.5 parts) rose to the blend of the 3 Tbsp tulsi and 2 Tbsp mimosa. This results in just under half a cup. When making a cup of tea with this blend, you would use 1-2 tsps of the final blend for an 8 oz cup.

35

Blend a Tea for Sleep Support

Teas have been used for centuries to help people fall asleep and stay asleep, resulting in thousands of different blends. When it comes to sleep, it's important to take into account the cause of sleep issues. Many people struggle with racing minds before bed, incontinence, or digestive issues, like heartburn. Combining herbs that can help with these issues, as well as sedative herbs, can make a powerful blend.

Common sedative herbs to consider: chamomile, lavender, California poppy, wild lettuce, valerian, catnip, ashwagandha, hops, linden, passionflower, and mimosa.

Create a dried herb blend with the proportions discussed on day 34 (3 parts base, 1-2 parts supporting herbs, and 1/4-1 parts accent herbs). Use the space to record your blend, its characteristics, and its flavor.

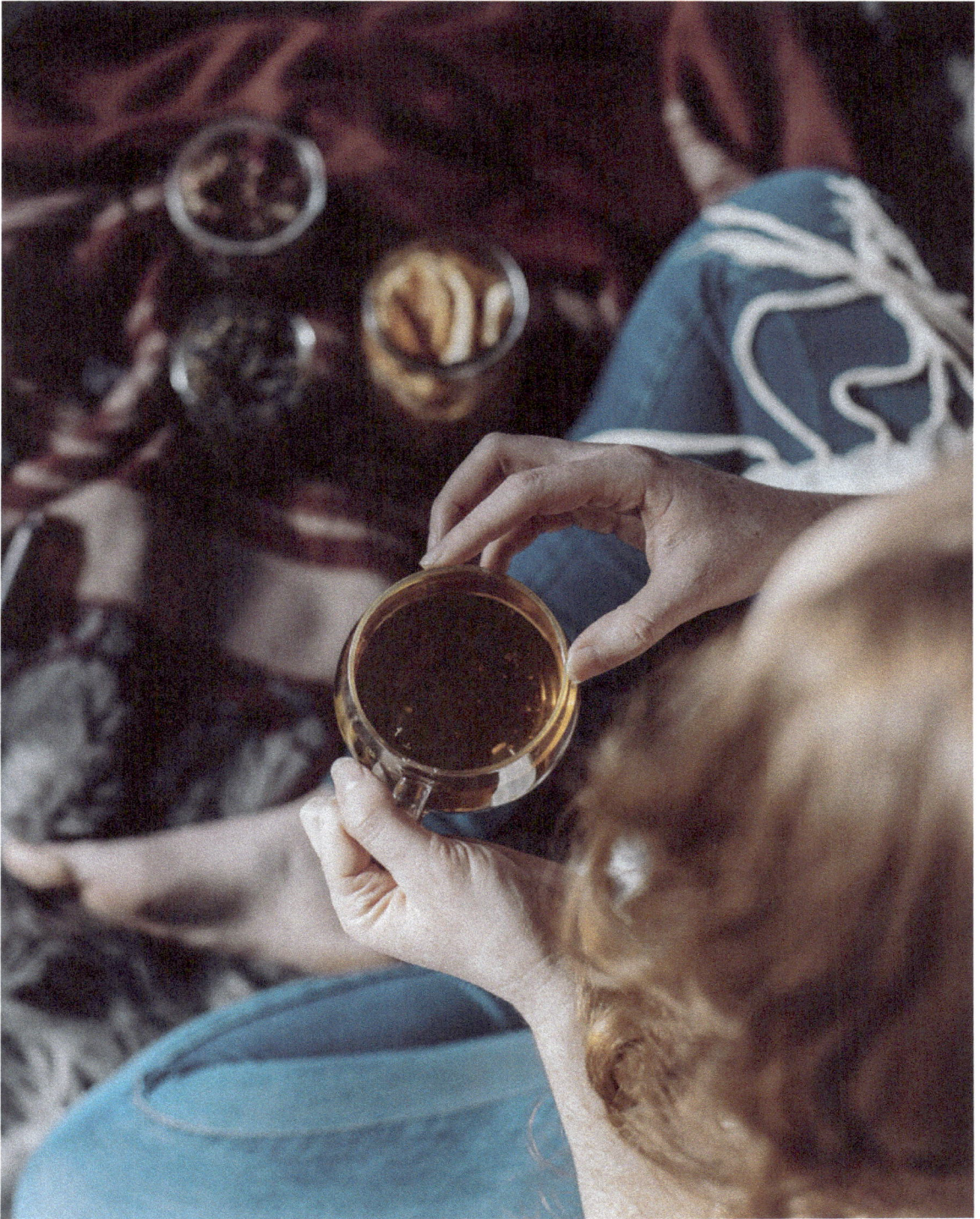

Simmer Pots

Simmer pots are an age-old classic, used for centuries to freshen homes and to cover unpleasant smells before scented candles were an option. They have a history of being used to cleanse and protect the air of the home and it's inhabitants. Many herbs have antimicrobial properties that can be aerosolized and carried throughout the home via simmer pots.

Simply add fragrant herbs, spices, and fruits to a pot of water and allow to simmer. Add additional water as needed.

Note: If left unattended, the pot can run out of water and scorch the bottom.

Floral Simmer Pot

Rose, lavender, thyme, lime slices

Fall Spice Simmer Pot

Cinnamon, nutmeg, cloves, orange slice, quartered apple

Fresh Air Simmer Pot

Lavender, eucalyptus, rosemary

Winter Hygge Simmer Pot

Pine, lemon, cranberry, cinnamon, clove

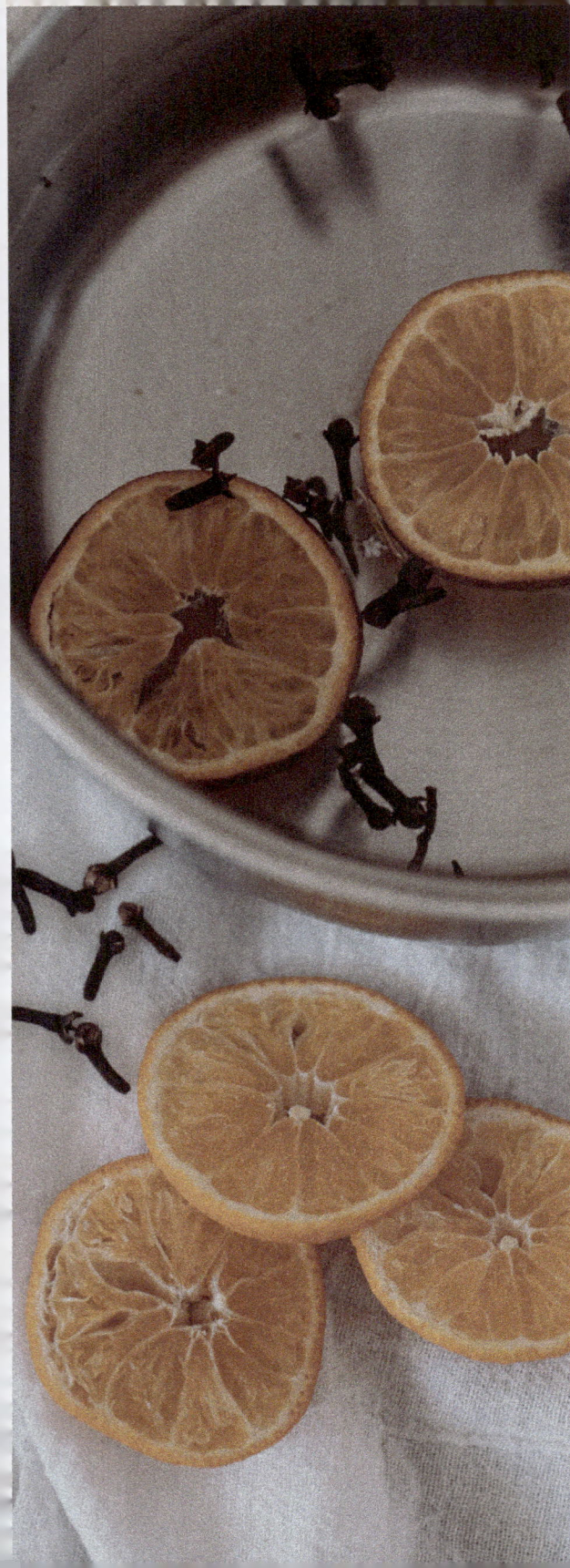

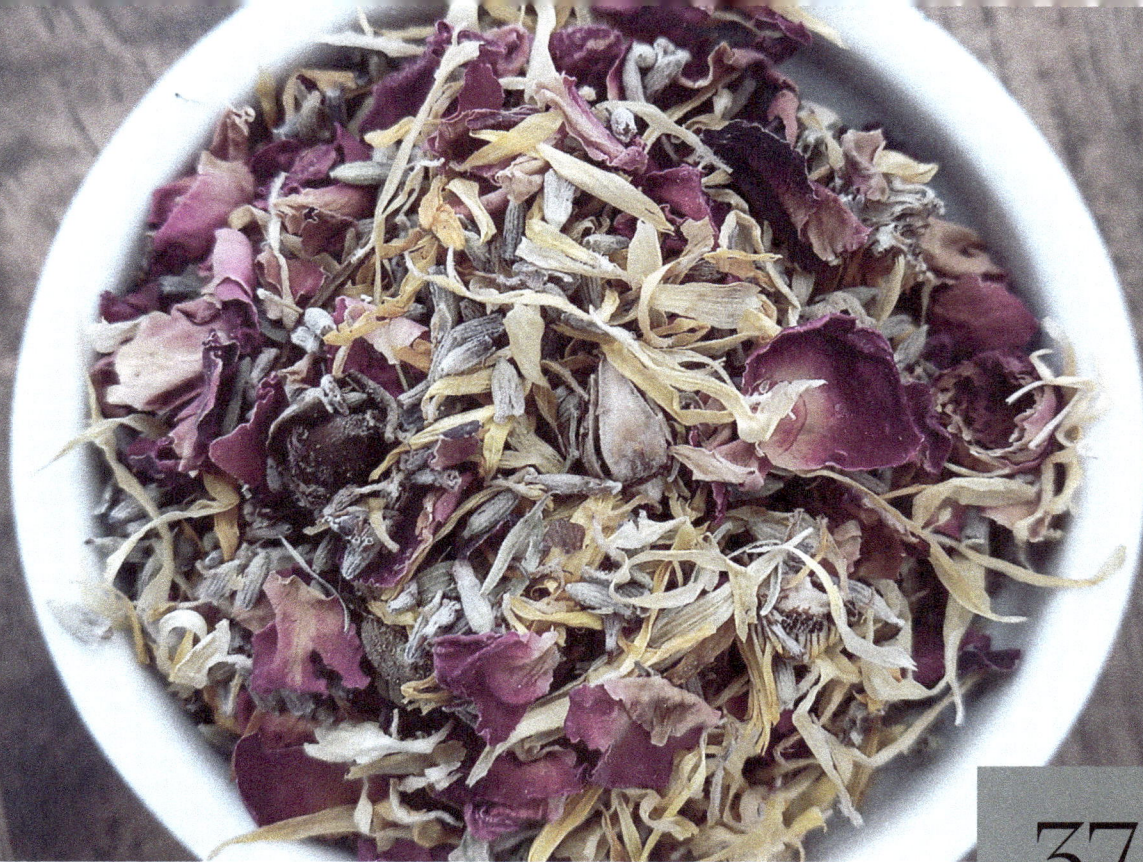

Herbal Face Steam

Herbal facial steams are an easy way to open pores and help remove impurities from the skin. They increase circulation, brighten complexion, and deeply hydrate the skin. Regularly using facial steams before cleansing and moisturizing can have incredible benefits.

1 cup boiling water
2-3 Tbsp dried herbs

Place herbs in a heat proof bowl or mug, and pour boiling water over top.

Position head over bowl, with closed eyes, and drape a towel over to create a tent and hold in the steam.

Remain tented for 5-10 minutes.

Look to day 26 for more information on herbs for skin care. Common blends to try:

Acne Blend
Lavender, rosemary, calendula, clove

Dry Skin Blend
Chamomile, lavender, rose, fennel

Oily Skin Blend
Lavender, peppermint, sage

Anti-Aging Blend
Rosemary, green tea, rose, lemon peel

Make your Own Spice Mixes

Using herbs in cooking is one of the easiest ways to incorporate extra medicinals into your life. Feeling a cold coming on? Make an immune boosting soup flavored with Italian seasoning. Have inflammation? Try a Massaman curry. Want to improve digestion? Opt for Moroccan spices.

Italian
2 Tbsp basil
2 Tbsp oregano
1 Tbsp red pepper
1 1/2 Tbsp garlic powder
1 Tbsp thyme
1 Tbsp rosemary
1/2 tsp onion powder
1/2 tsp sea salt

Taco
2 Tbsp ground cumin
1 1/2 tsp paprika
1 tsp garlic powder
1/2 tsp onion powder
1/2 tsp cayenne pepper
1 /2 tsp chili powder
1/4 tsp sea salt
1/4 tsp ground pepper
1/4 tsp oregano

Ranch
2 Tbsp dried parsley
1 Tbsp dried chives
1/2 Tbsp garlic powder
1 tsp onion powder
1 tsp dried dill
1 tsp salt
1/2 tsp ground pepper

Cajun
2 Tbsp ground cumin
2 Tbsp coriander
2 Tbsp paprika
2 tsp oregano
1 1/2 tsp salt
1 1/2 tsp ground pepper
1 1/4-2 tsp cayenne

Curry
2 Tbsp cumin, toasted
2 Tbsp tsp coriander
1 1/2 Tbsp turmeric
2 tsp salt
2 tsp ground ginger
1 tsp ground mustard
1/2 tsp black pepper
1/2 tsp cardamom
1/2 tsp cinnamon
cayenne to taste

Moroccan
1 tsp ground cumin
1 tsp ground ginger
1 tsp salt
3/4 tsp black pepper
1/2 tsp ground cinnamon
1/2 tsp ground coriander
1/2 tsp cayenne
1/2 tsp ground allspice
1/4 tsp ground cloves

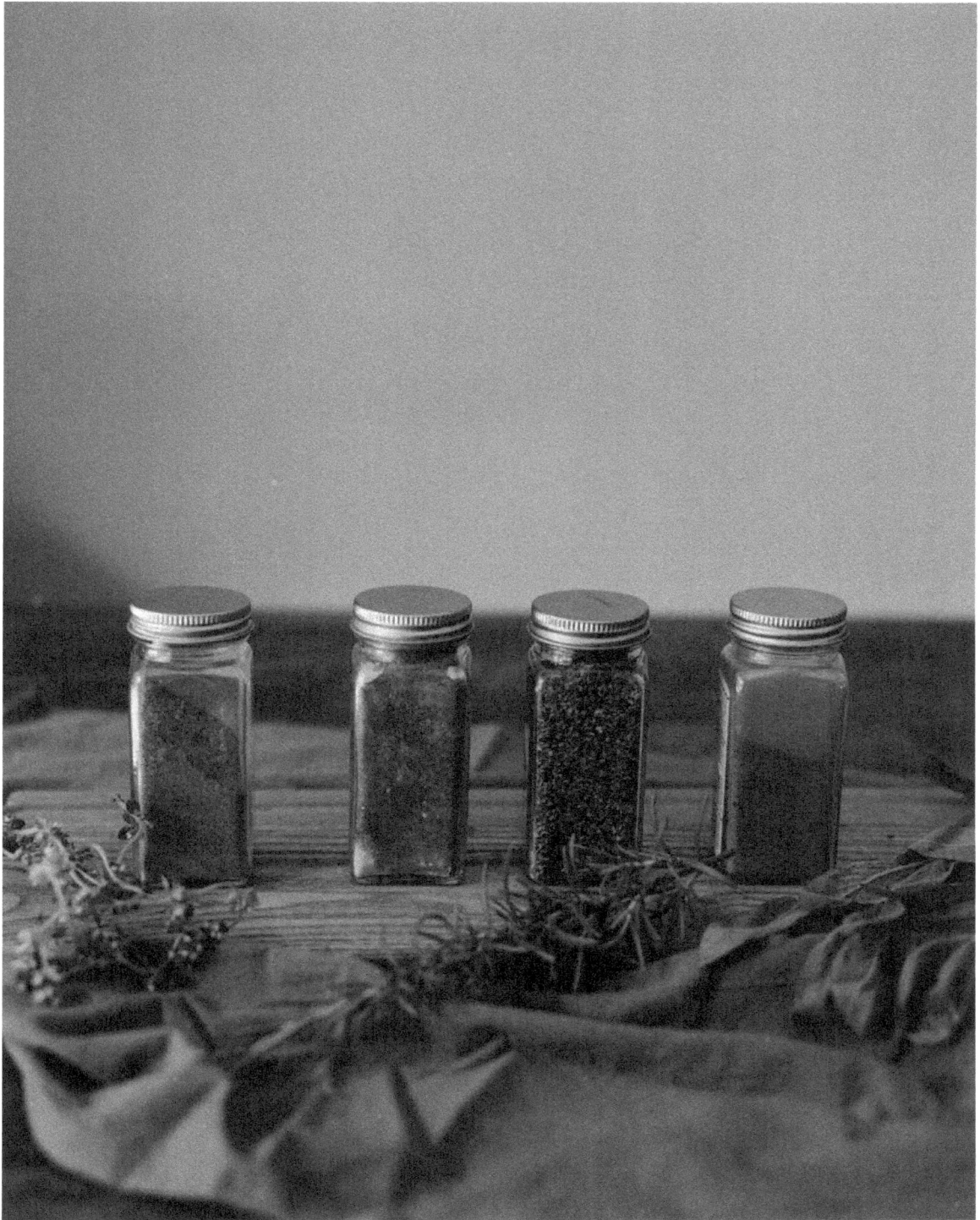

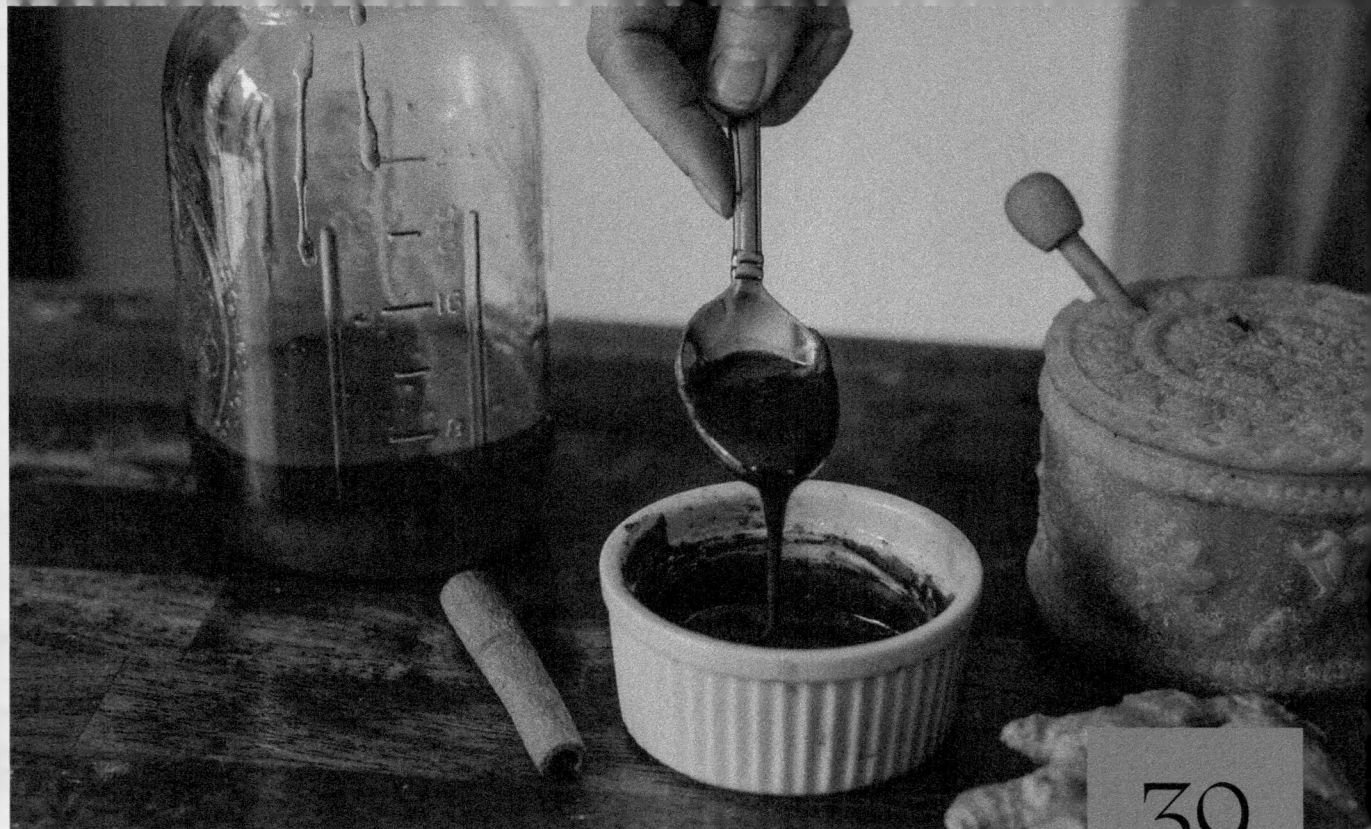

Make an Electuary

Electuaries are a great alternative for those who truly don't like the taste of many herbal preparations. Made by combining powdered herb (discussed on day 27) and honey, the sweetness of the honey cuts the bitterness from the herbs, making them more palatable. Electuaries can be added to drinks (1-2 tsp per 8 oz liquid), spread on toast, pastries, or used as a treat.

1 part powdered herb
1-2 parts honey

Combine powdered herbs and honey in a clean jar, stirring until well combined.

Seal and store for 6-12 months. Electuaries with a higher honey content can last longer. Discard if mold appears.

The dosage for most powdered herbs is 2-6 grams, or 1-2 tsp, 1-3 times daily. Keep this in mind when using electuaries medicinally.

Common blend to try:

Sore Throat Blend
Licorice root, ginger, cinnamon

Sleep & Nerves
Lemon balm, chamomile, pinch of salt

Electrolyte Blend
Hibiscus, lemon balm, nettle, pinch of salt
(add a few drops lemon when serving)

Easy Herbal Pill Balls

This old-fashioned method of making herbal pills is a great way to get your daily herbs. However, it is difficult to get an exact volume of herbal material in each pill. It is not recommended if specific dosing is needed (in the case of an infection) or if over-use is a concern. This is a great way to utilize adaptogens, nervine, or nutritive herbs, especially for kids or while traveling.

Nutritive Herb Balls
2 Tbsp dandelion root powder
1 tsp alfalfa powder
1 tsp burdock root powder
honey or maple syrup
cocoa or cinnamon powder as needed

Combine powdered herbs in a bowl. Add honey or syrup in teaspoon increments until a thick, sticky paste forms.

In the same fashion, add small amounts of cocoa or cinnamon while stirring until a dough is formed. Knead the dough. Form small balls, roughly 1/2 tsp in size or a size that can easily be swallowed.

Place the balls on a cookie sheet, and set in the oven at as low of a temperature as the oven allows. Dehydrate the pill balls until they are firm all the way through (about 1 hour).

Note: You can also use one of the blends from day 39.

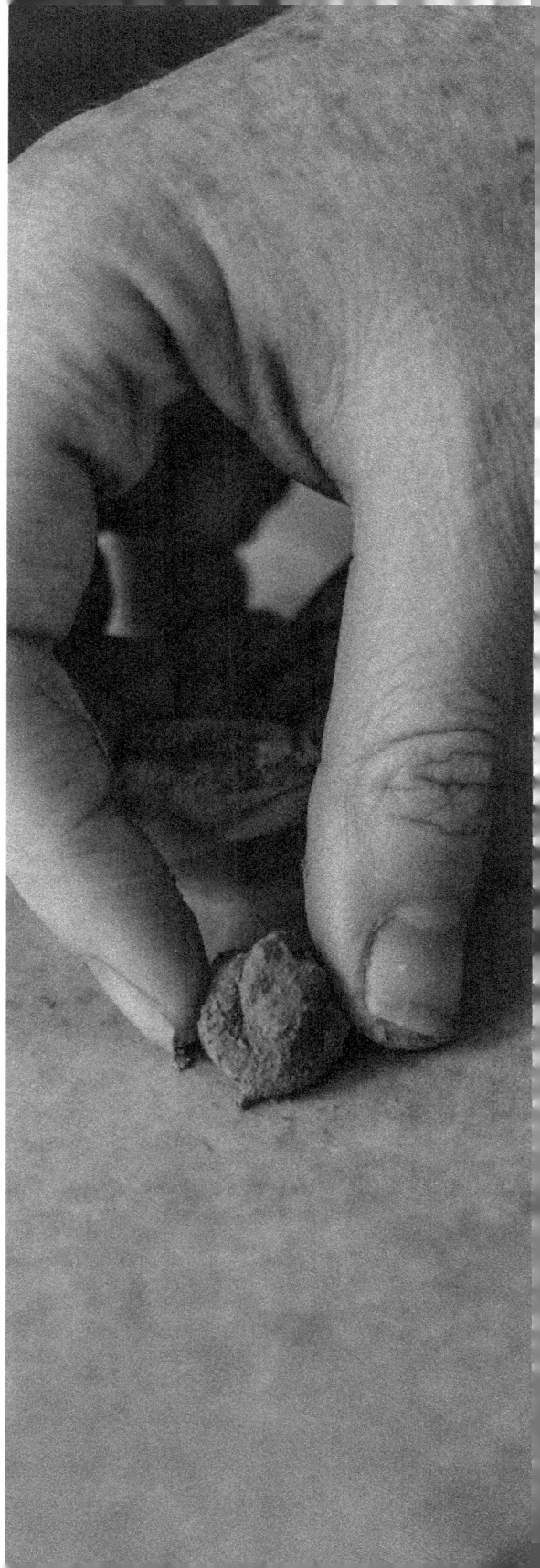

What Taste Can Tell Us About Herbs

Taste is one of our most powerful senses. Throughout our evolution as humans, our sense of taste has been able to help us identify foods that are potentially harmful, as well as foods that can benefit us in survival situations. When it comes to herbs, taste can help us identify the medicinal components and the actions of plants. Go back to day 17 to review herbal actions.

Most of us are familiar with the five basic flavors; sweet, salty, sour, bitter, and umami/pungent. Each of these flavors denotes different qualities and actions of herbs.

Sweet

A well-loved flavor – sweetness in an herb usually signifies toning, which calm, moisten, and nourish. They tend to have anti-inflammatory, often demulcent, and sometimes adaptogenic actions. Examples: licorice, burdock, marshmallow, milky oats, and astragulus.

Salty

Salty herbs are often linked to those with high mineral content. The flavor denotes herbs that are highly nourishing, restorative, and typically diuretic. Examples: nettle, oatstraw, cleavers, chickweed, violet, and seaweeds.

Sour

Herbs that are sour will usually cleanse tissues, cool tissues, and improve mineral absorption. While some herbal traditions (like Ayurveda) categorize sour and astringent flavors separately, sour herbs still tend to have the astringent quality. Sour herbs are usually high in tannins, which are known to pull moisture inward. This can be useful in cases of diarrhea, bleeding, or damp/relaxation states. Examples: oregano, hibiscus, fermented foods, rose, hawthorn, sage.

Bitter

Humans have evolved along side of plants, allowing us to utilize many of them in a very unique way. Bitterness tends to be a sign of toxic substances plants create to protect themselves from potential threats. In order to protect ourselves from these substances, our bodies have adapted to stimulate bile production, improve digestion, and eliminate these toxins from the body when the bitter taste receptors are activated. This effectively allows us to break down the toxins while still retain the plant nutrients. Examples: rhubarb, motherwort, dandelion, gentian, dark leafy greens, artichoke, coffee, and tea.

Pungent

Also associated with spicy or stimulating flavors. These herbs are generally stimulating, especially for the digestion and metabolism. They tend to be very aromatic, anti-microbial, and help promote circulation and sweating. Examples: ginger, garlic, rosemary, pepper, cayenne, thyme, oregano, cuman, juniper, horseradish, and clove.

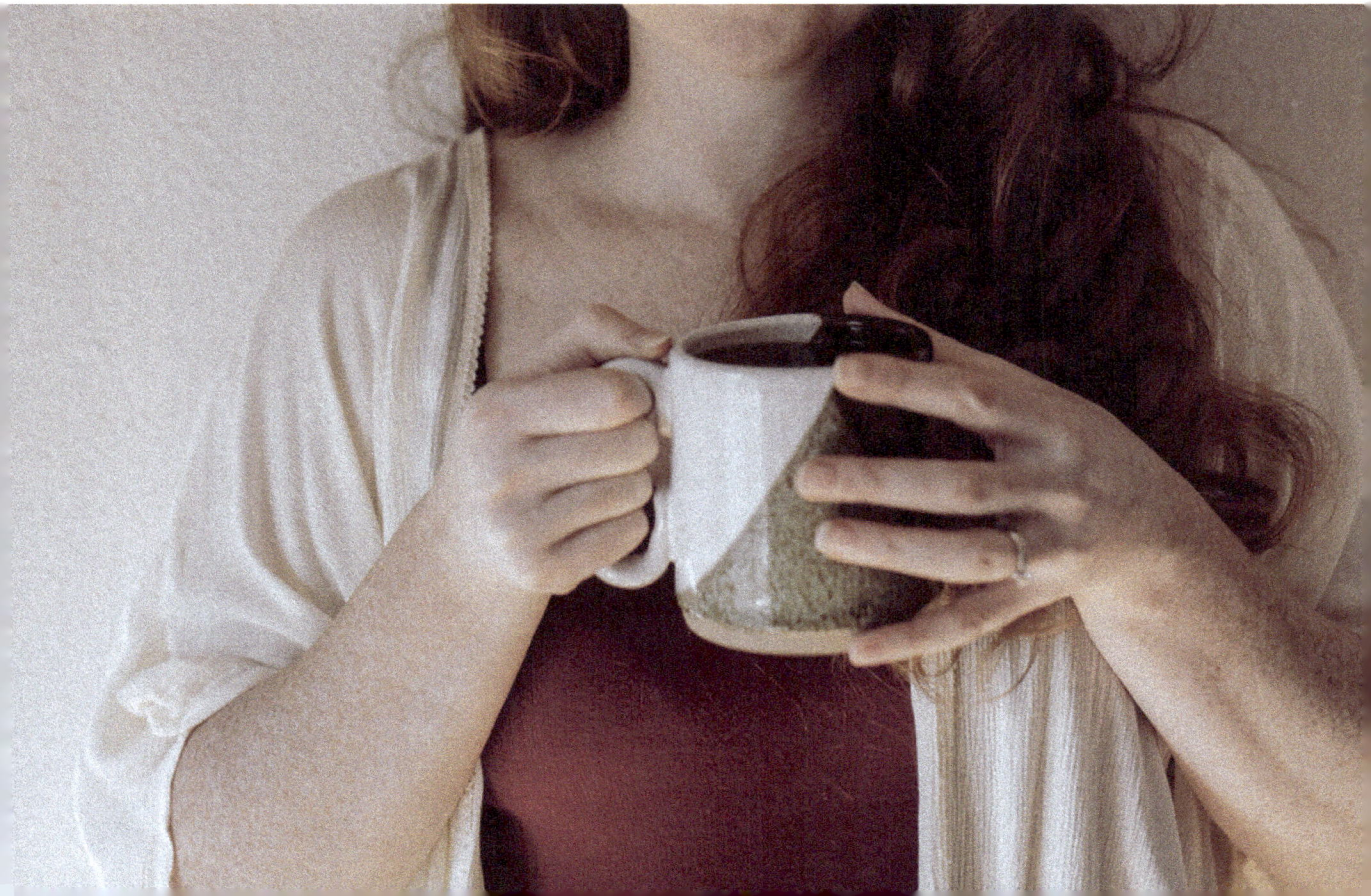

Tastes & Actions Activity

Fill in the boxes with herbs with their corresponding action listed on the right. Take note of some of the herbs we have already used such as chamomile, nettle, mint, tulsi, hibiscus, ashwaganda, and more. Review the information on herbal actions from day 17 and throughout the book. Try to draw connections between previous experiences with the herbs and with the knowledge you have gained.

Herb	Flavor	Actions
Ginger	Pungent	Anodyne (painkiller), Anti-inflammatory, Anti-microbial, Anti-spasmodic, Carminative, Circulatory Stimulant, Choleretic, Diaphoretic, expectorant

43

Herbal Pillows

There is a long history of using herbs throughout the home or under a pillow to protect against evil, to bring good dreams, luck, love, to heal illness, and more. In modern day, we know that something as simple as the scent of certain plants can trigger responses in the body and even change our moods. Create a relaxing herbal pillow to place under your own or to carry for comfort is a great way to keep this tradition alive.

Additionally, herbal pillows can be tossed in drawers or musty closets to help ward off unwanted pests (spiders and mice will avoid mint), or to freshen up a space. The addition of salts can help absorb moisture, and prevent mildew.

Making an herbal pillow can be as simple as filling a muslin bag with herbs and essential oils, securing the opening closed, or as complicated as sewing a small pillow enclosed with the herbs and oils.

Larger pillows are often sewn with dried rice or beans in them, as well as herbs. The rice and beans allow the pillows to retain heat, and be used for warming a bed, soothing sore muscles, or assisting with headaches.

Suggested blends to help you get started:

Sweet Sleep
Rose, lavender, catnip, chamomile, lemon balm

Uplifting Mint
Lemon verbena, peppermint, eucalyptus

WoodlandDreams
Cedar, pine, geranium, lavender, sage, rose, orange

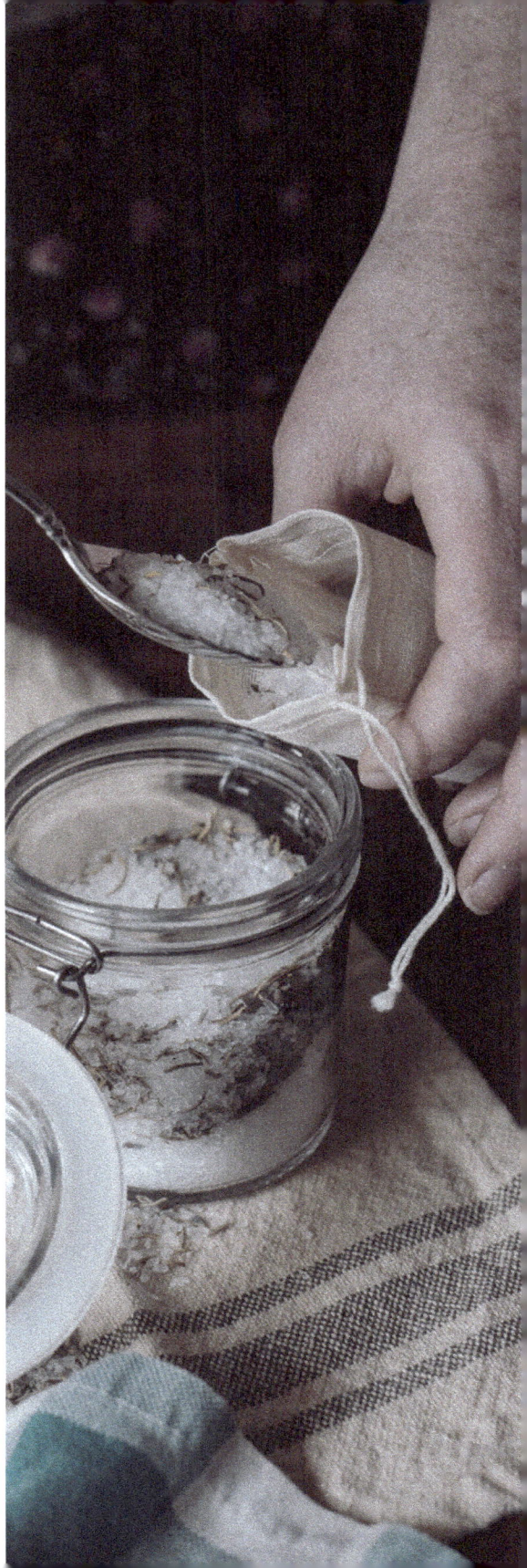

Rose Water

Rose water has been used for centuries for health, and beauty. You can find rose water used in beauty treatments, as well as perfume. It's well known to soothe irritation, calm redness, repair skin damage, and ease skin conditions, like acne, eczema, psoriasis, and rosacea. Medicinally, it has been shown to benefit eye health, digestion, brain health, as well as fight infection, headaches, and sore throat.

While there are several methods for making rosewater, we are going to use the steam method. Steaming results in one of the most potent products. Other methods include distillation, and a simple tea infusion.

Rose Water Steam Method

2 cups fresh organic rose petals
1 cup ice cubes
1/2 gallon distilled water

Place a small heat resistant bowl in the center of a wide pot. Place the petals around the bowl in the pan. Add distilled water to the pan until petals are just submerged. Be sure the rim of the bowl remains above water.

Place a lid upside down on the pot, and place the ice cubes on top.

Heat the entire set over medium-high heat, bringing to a low simmer. The steam from the simmering rose petals will hit the cool top and drip into the bowl via the tops handle.

Continue simmering until the petals have lost their color. Remove from heat and let cool.

Remove the bowl and pour into a sealable jar.

Store in the fridge for up to 6 months.

The leftover rose petals and water from the pan can be used as a rose infusion, but it will not be as potent as the steamed liquid. This infusion will only last 3-5 days in the fridge.

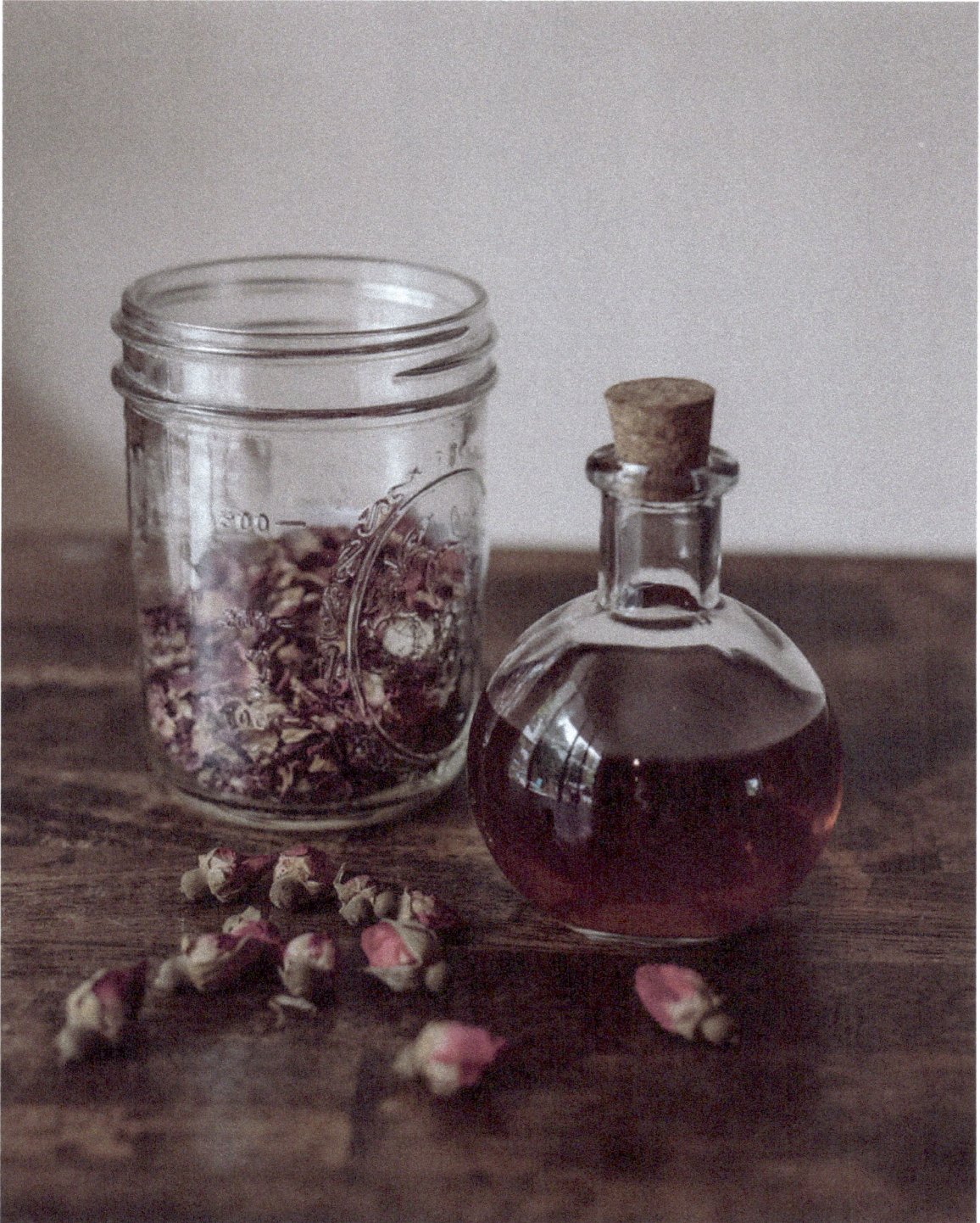

45

Make a Ginger Bug

A ginger bug is a slurry of fresh ginger, sugar, and water that has been allowed to ferment until bubbly and foamy. It is used as the base for probiotic and naturally bubbly drinks, such as sodas, herbal beers, and tonics. Naturally fermented drinks are not only a wonderful treat, but have the health benefit of supporting digestion, metabolism, and immune strength. Turn to day 50 for suggested recipes and decanting.

Day 1
2 cups water
2 tsp sugar
1 oz fresh ginger, diced

Warm the water and sugar in a pan over medium heat, until sugar is fully dissolved and liquid mixture is clear. Remove from heat and allow to cool completely.

Combine room temperature sugar water and ginger in a pint jar. Seal and set in a cool dark place.

Day 2-5
5 tsp sugar
2 ½ oz fresh ginger, diced

The next day (2), stir in 1 tsp sugar and additional 1/2 oz ginger into the jar. Seal and set in a cool dark place.

Repeat steps form day 2 on days 3, 4, and 5. The mixture will begin to bubble and smell like yeast.

If after day five, the mixture has not reached desired fermentation, continue to repeat step 2 for an additional 1-3 days.

Combine 1/2 cup ginger bug with fruit juice or sweetened herbal tea. Bottle as desired, and let ferment for 3 days.

Move to the fridge to slow down fermentation. Drink within 1-2 weeks.

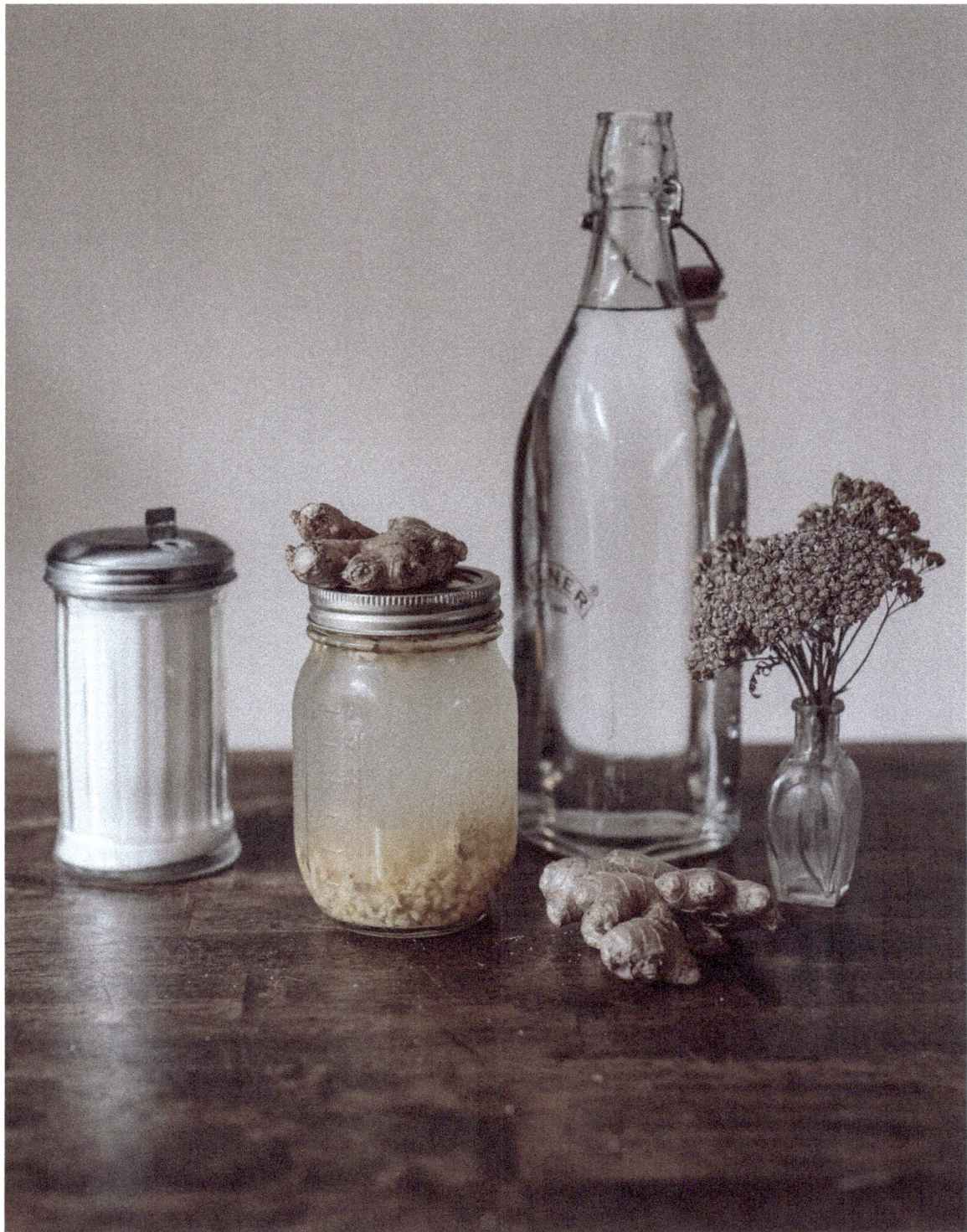

Culinary Herbal Salts

Herbal salts are one of the easiest ways to add flavor and intrigue to your daily meals, while providing nutrients and herbal benefits.

Combining herbs for a specific purpose allows for utilization of a salt in small doses throughout the day. This multiplies herbal benefits, including increased nutrient absorption, reduced inflammation, and emotional support.

To create herbal salts, combine equal parts powdered herb and ground salt of choice. Use a coffee grinder to power herbs (see day 27 for details on powdering herbs).

Mineral Blend

1 part nettle
1 part alfalfa
1 part spirulina
3 parts table salt

Adaptogen Blend

1 part reishi
1 part chaga
1 part cordyceps
1 part shiitake
4 parts himalayan salt

Inflammation Blend

2 parts turmeric
2 parts nettle
1 part ginger
5 parts sea salt

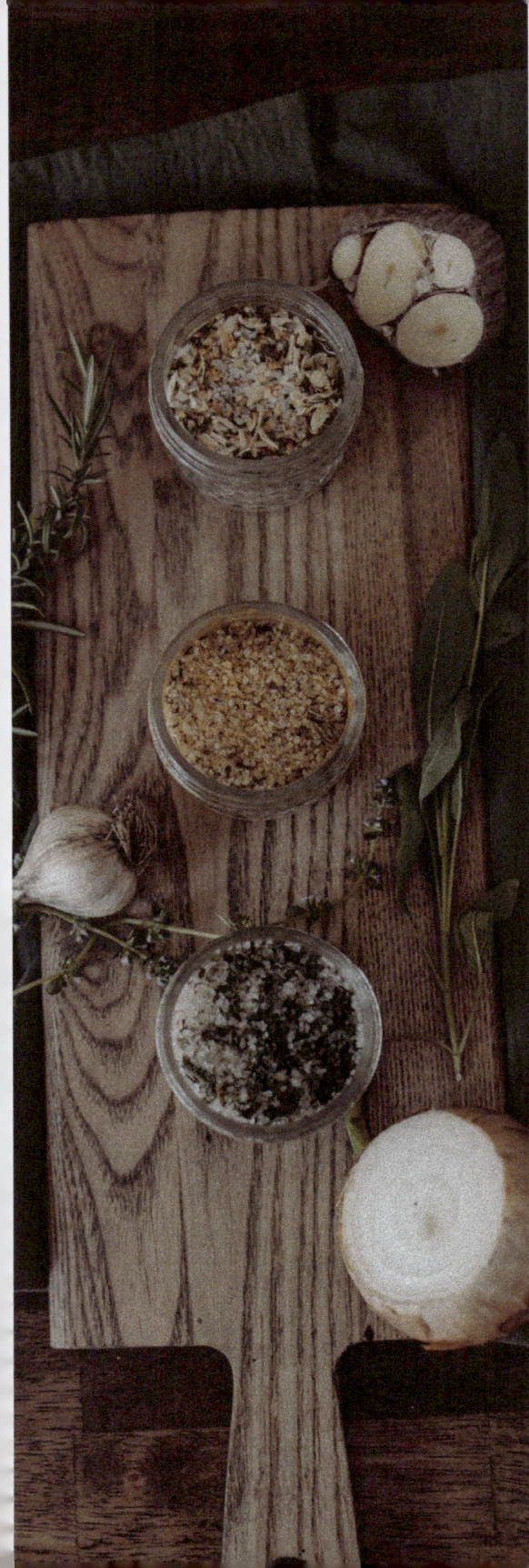

Make Bitters

Bitters are an alcohol extraction of bitter herbs. When our taste buds signal that the bitter flavor is present, it triggers our body to prepare for digestion. Bile and digestive enzymes are secreted into the stomach, and mucus is made in the digestive tract. Using bitters on a regular basis has been shown to improve nutrient absorption, naturally detox the liver, improve immune function, reduce heartburn, gas, and bloating. They have even been shown to improve stress response.

Some bitter herbs include: gentian, dandelion, burdock, oregon grape, chamomile, artichoke leaf, citrus peel, milk thistle, chicory root, wild cherry bark, and sarsaparilla.

This recipe is an adaption of the ever-popular Angostura Bitters commonly used today in bars and restaurants, and even found in grocery stores.

Spiced Bitters

0.3 oz dried dandelion
0.2 oz dried ginger
0.2 oz dried gentian root
0.2 oz dried orange peel
0.1 oz dried clove
5 oz of 180 proof alcohol (by volume)

Combine herbs and alcohol in a sterile mason jar, securing with a paper lined lid.

Place in a dark cabinet and allow to infuse for 6-8 weeks, shaking occasionally.

Look to day 86 and 87 for straining and use instructions

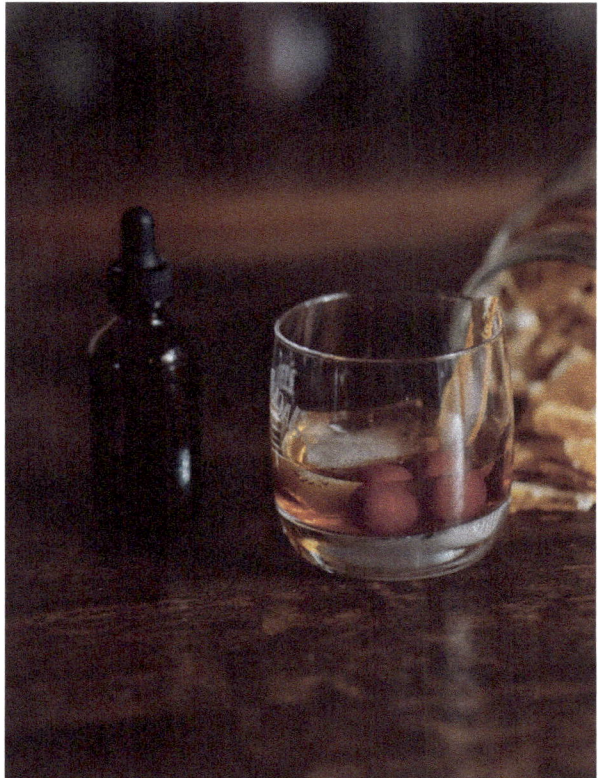

48

Berry Sage & Skullcap Shrub

Shrubs are a type of drinking vinegar made with sugar, as opposed to oxymels that are made with honey (described on day 11). This particular recipe utilizes heat to help infuse the herbs and fruit. The shrub will also only infuse for 24-36 hours. This method provides an abundance of flavor, as well as medicinal benefits. Perfect for a relaxing, evening sip.

1 cup fresh raspberries
1 cup sugar
1.5 Tbsp dried sage
2.5 Tbsp dried skullcap
1 cup raw apple cider vinegar

In a small saucepan, combine berries and sugar over medium heat. Bring to a simmer, stirring regularly for 5-6 minutes, or until the berries begin to break down and mixture thickens.

Remove from heat, add herbs and vinegar. Let cool completely before placing in fridge overnight (up to 36 hours).

Strain mixture and serve 1-2 oz with ice and seltzer or water.

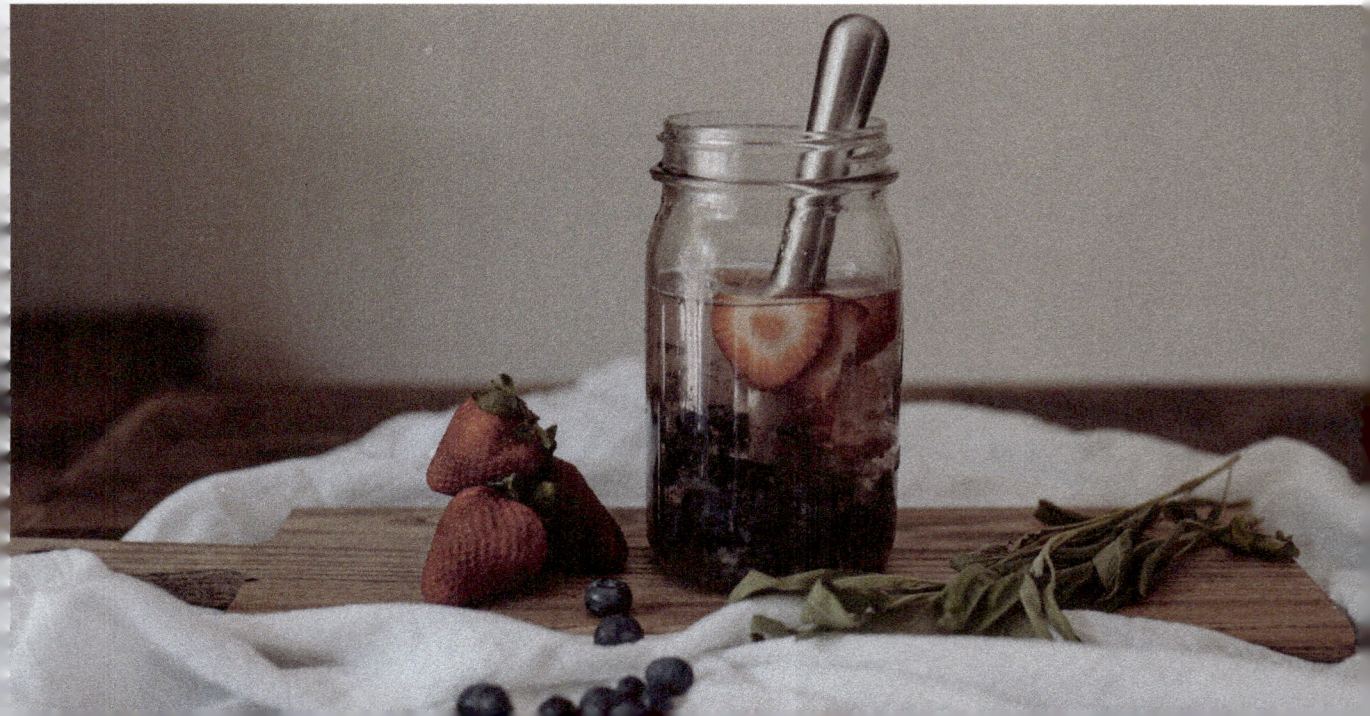

Fermented Honey

Fermented honey is a great way to preserve herbs. It's also a tasty way to administer them. Because honey is full of wild yeast, it will ferment easily with only a small amount of moisture added. Fresh herbs typically have enough water in them to begin the fermentation process.

This particular recipe utilizes garlic and ginger for their immune-boosting power. While the combination may sound spicy, the fermentation process will remove much of the bite, resulting in a mellow and sweet overall flavor.

Honeyed Ginger & Garlic

2 heads garlic, peeled
1/3 cup fresh ginger, sliced
1 cup raw honey

Combine herbs in a sterile jar. You can choose to mince the garlic and ginger, but it is not necessary. Pour in honey and seal the jar. Invert a few times to be sure the herbs are coated. Loosen the lid just enough to let some gas to escape as necessary.

Place in a cool dark area for roughly 4 weeks. Give the jar a light shake every couple of days. Fermentation should begin in a few days. The mixture can be used at any point in the process.

Use 1 Tbsp 2x daily as an immune booster.

Note: Fermented honey can be used to create sauces and salad dressings. They can be used in cooking, but heat will kill off any beneficial bacteria, however medicinal benefits will be present.

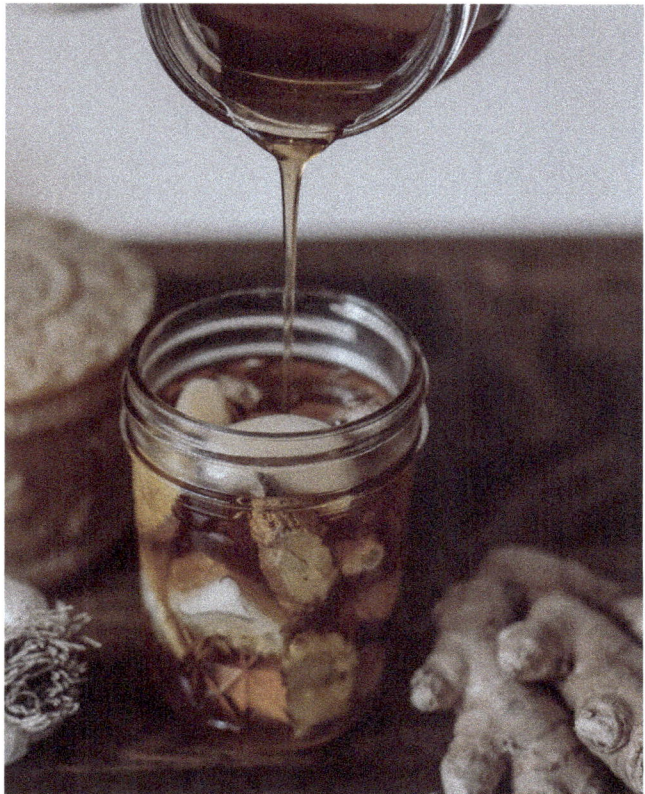

Homemade Ginger Ale

There are several ways to make a basic ginger ale. However, this fermented version is one of the healthiest. Not only does it contain the many benefits of ginger, but also contains the gut health benefits of natural probiotics. Most of the sugar is used up during fermentation – resulting in a sweet-tasting, low sugar drink. It's easy to add additional herbs and flavors during the first steps of this recipe, while increasing the health benefits.

Fermented Ginger Ale

4 cups filtered water
1/3 cup sugar
2-3 inch piece of fresh ginger root, sliced thin
1/4 cup ginger bug starter (day 45)
Splash lemon or lime juice (optional)

Combine water, fresh ginger and sugar in a pot, bringing to a boil. Reduce heat to a simmer, and continue to cook for 4-5 minutes.

Remove from heat and allow to cool to room temperature. Strain into a quart-sized glass jar.

Use a wooden spoon to stir in the ginger bug and lemon or lime juice, and seal.

Let ferment for 3-6 days, opening the jar every 1-2 days so that it does not build up too much carbonation.

The ginger ale is done fermenting – when the liquid will be fizzy, and slightly sweet. If it is still too sweet, allow to continue fermentation; testing it every 1-2 days until the desired flavor is achieved.

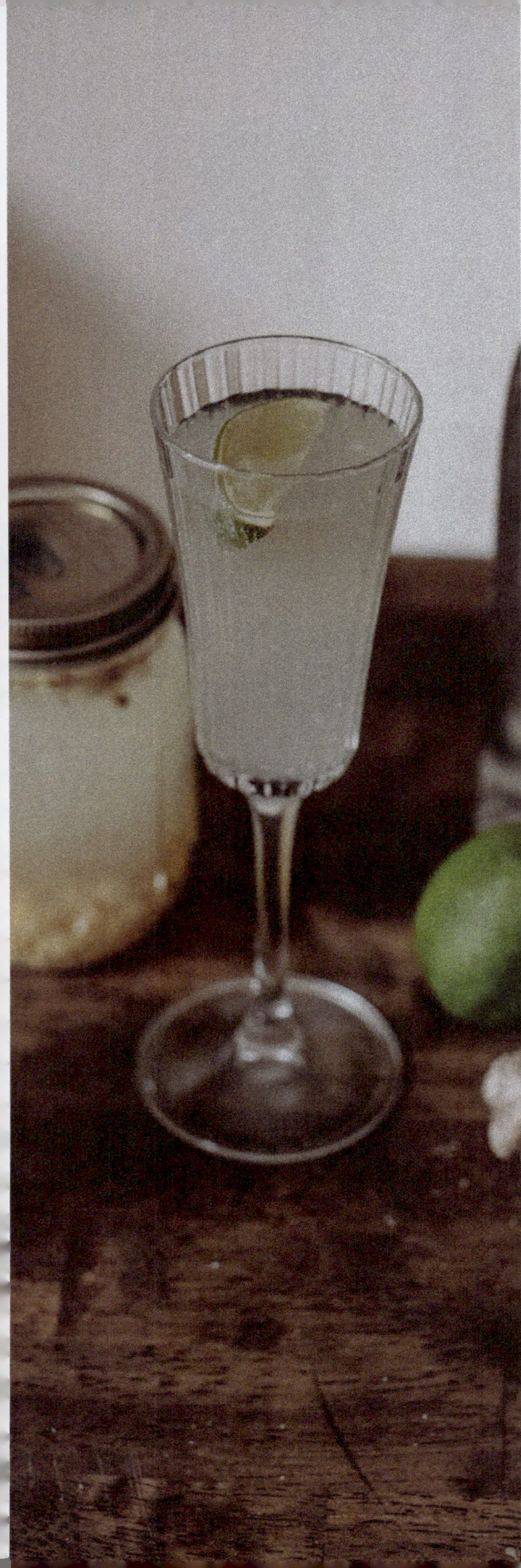

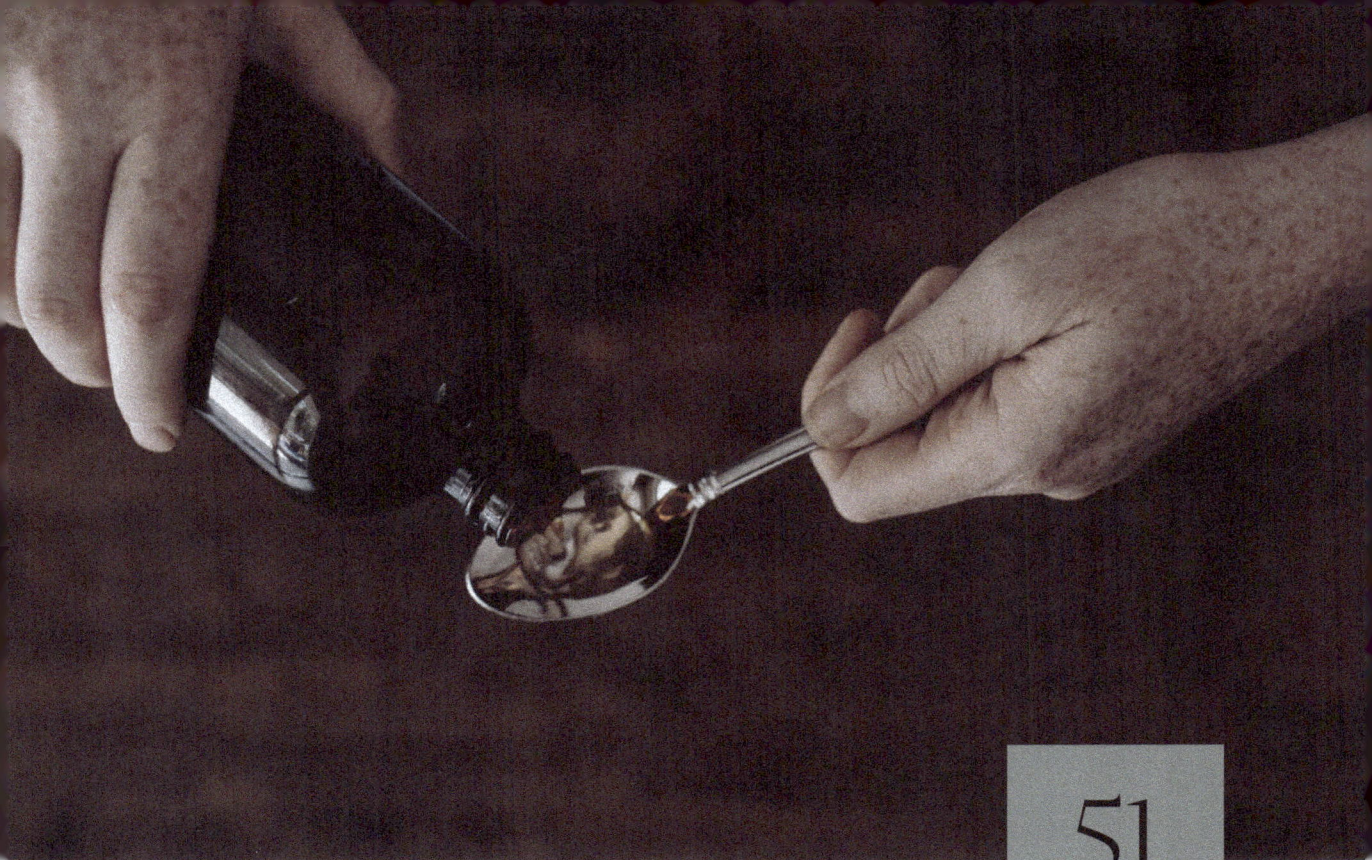

Easy Clove Mouthwash

Cloves have anti-fungal, anti-bacterial, analgesic, and anti-inflammatory properties. This means that cloves can fight bad breath and bacteria in the mouth, while also being able to aid in reducing gum swelling, irritation, and soothing toothaches. Cloves can enhance circulation in the mouth, improving overall gum health.

Combine this clove mouthwash with additional immune boosting herbs, such as echinacea or mint for pain and fresh breath, cinnamon, or sage to help prevent plaque and improve overall oral health.

1 cup water
1 tsp whole cloves

Bring water to a boil in a small pan.

Place whole cloves in a heat-resistant container, such as a mason jar.

Carefully pour boiling water over cloves.

Cover the container and allow mixture to cool (20-30 minutes).

Strain mouthwash and pour into a clean container with a lid.

Use as you would any mouthwash. Do not swallow.

52

Herbal Massage Oil

Use the herbal oil blend that was prepared by slow infusion on day 12 to create your own relaxing massage oil. After 4-6 weeks of infusing, your oil should be slightly darker in color. Some herbs will change the color of the oil more than others. It should still smell neutral and slightly herbaceous. If the blend smells moldy, rancid, or has visible mold, discard it and start over.

To strain, line a fine mesh sieve with cheesecloth, and pour the infusion through. Use the cheesecloth to squeeze out as much oil as possible. Discard the herbs, and pour the final oil into a sterile jar. If there is a lot of sediment present, you may need to strain again, slowly with a coffee filter.

Once strained, you should be left with just over 1 cup of infused oil. Be sure to reserve at least 1/2 cup for the activity on day 53. The recipe below outlines how to create an aromatic massage oil. While essential oils are not necessary, they add both scent and medicinal qualities.

Calming essential oils include: lavender, rose, jasmine, ylang ylang, chamomile, cedarwood, and patchouli.

Herbal Massage Oil

1/2 cup of infused oil
6-7 drops vitamin E
25-30 drops essential oils (optional)

Combine all ingredients, stirring gently.

Add a small amount to the palm of the hands, and massage into skin as desired.

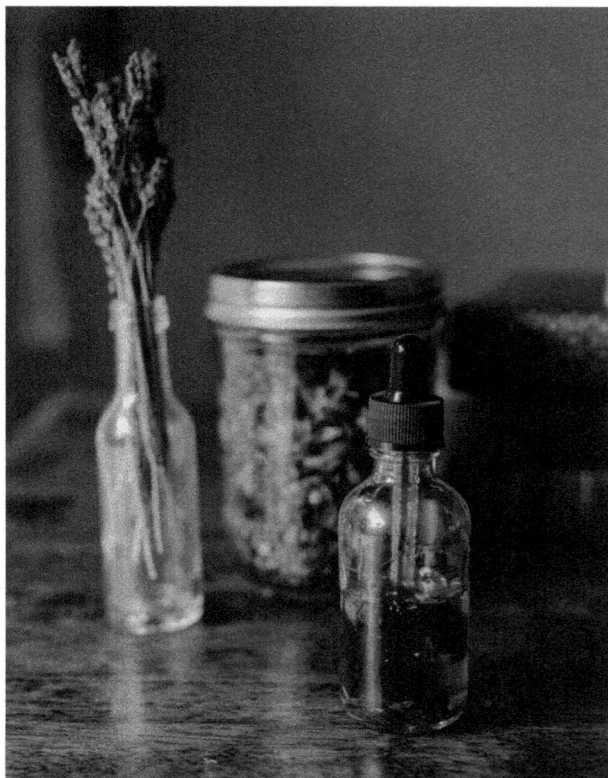

Make a Body Butter

Body butters are a classic way to utilize herbal infused oils as well as natural moisturizers, creating a luxurious skin-healing blend. The main difference between a body butter and usual creams and lotions is that body butter does not contain water-based ingredients (like hydrosols or aloe vera gel). This makes them shelf stable without preservatives or emulsifiers. This also makes them ultra-moisturizing to the skin.

Use the leftover oil from your long infused herbal blend (day 13), the heat method (day 23), or create your own using the information provided on day 12.

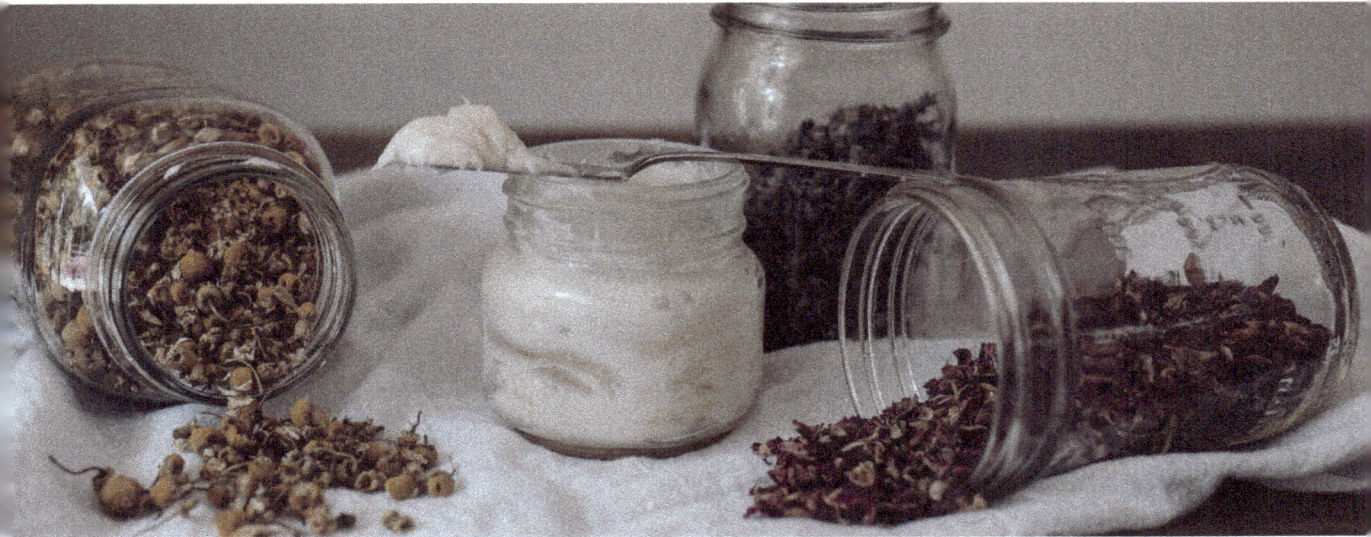

Whipped Body Butter

1 cup cocoa or shea butter
1/2 cup infused oil
2 Tbsp beeswax pellets
1 tsp arrow root powder (optional)
5 drops vitamin E oil (optional)
10 drops essential oils (optional)

Combine butters, oils, and wax in a double boiler over medium heat. Allow to melt completely, stirring occasionally.

Remove from heat and whisk in additional ingredients. Place in fridge to cool for 1 hour.

Once slightly cooled, the mixture should be mostly, but not completely, solid.

Use a hand mixer to whip for 10 minutes until fluffy.

Store in an air tight container in a cool, dark place for up to 6 months.

Herbal Broth

Broth has a long tradition of being an incredibly healthful food, and a cooking staple for centuries. Whether you prefer a bone or a vegetable broth, adding helpful herbs is a great way to increase both health potency and flavor.

For bone based broths, herbs can be added at the end of the process. With vegetable broths that only simmer for an hour or so, herbs can be added at the beginning. For either version, you may use a pre-made broth and simply follow the recipe below before use.

Basic Herbal Broth

6 cups broth of choice
3 dried bay leaves
1/2 cup fresh herbs of choice
2-4 garlic cloves
salt and pepper to taste

Combine all ingredients in a large stock pot. Bring to a simmer, stirring occasionally for 1-2 hours. Strain and use as desired.

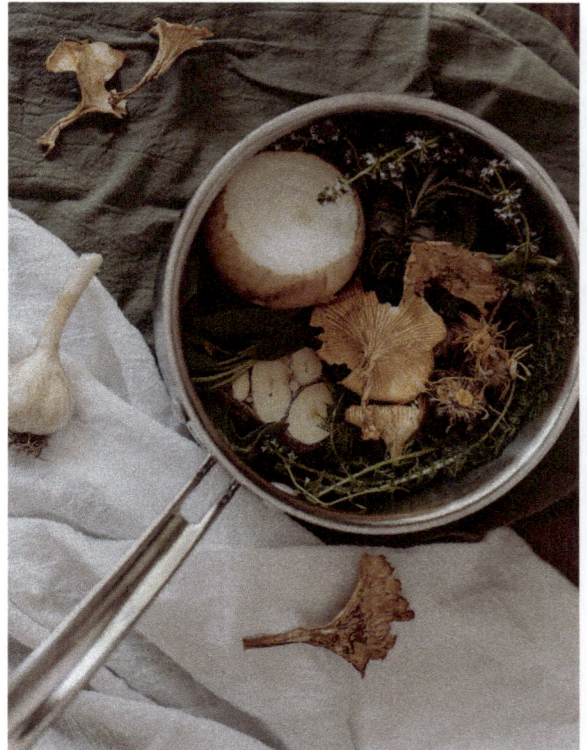

Herb Combinations

Thai Style - tulsi, lime, lemongrass, cilantro, ginger, cayenne

Mushroom Immune - shiitake, reishi, and Chaga mushrooms, astragalus root, sage, parsley

Anti-Inflammatory - turmeric, ginger, garlic, nettle, calendula

Cold Care - thyme, parsley, oregano, echinacea, sage, onion, lemon

Super Mineral - burdock root, dandelion root, nettle, shiitake mushrooms

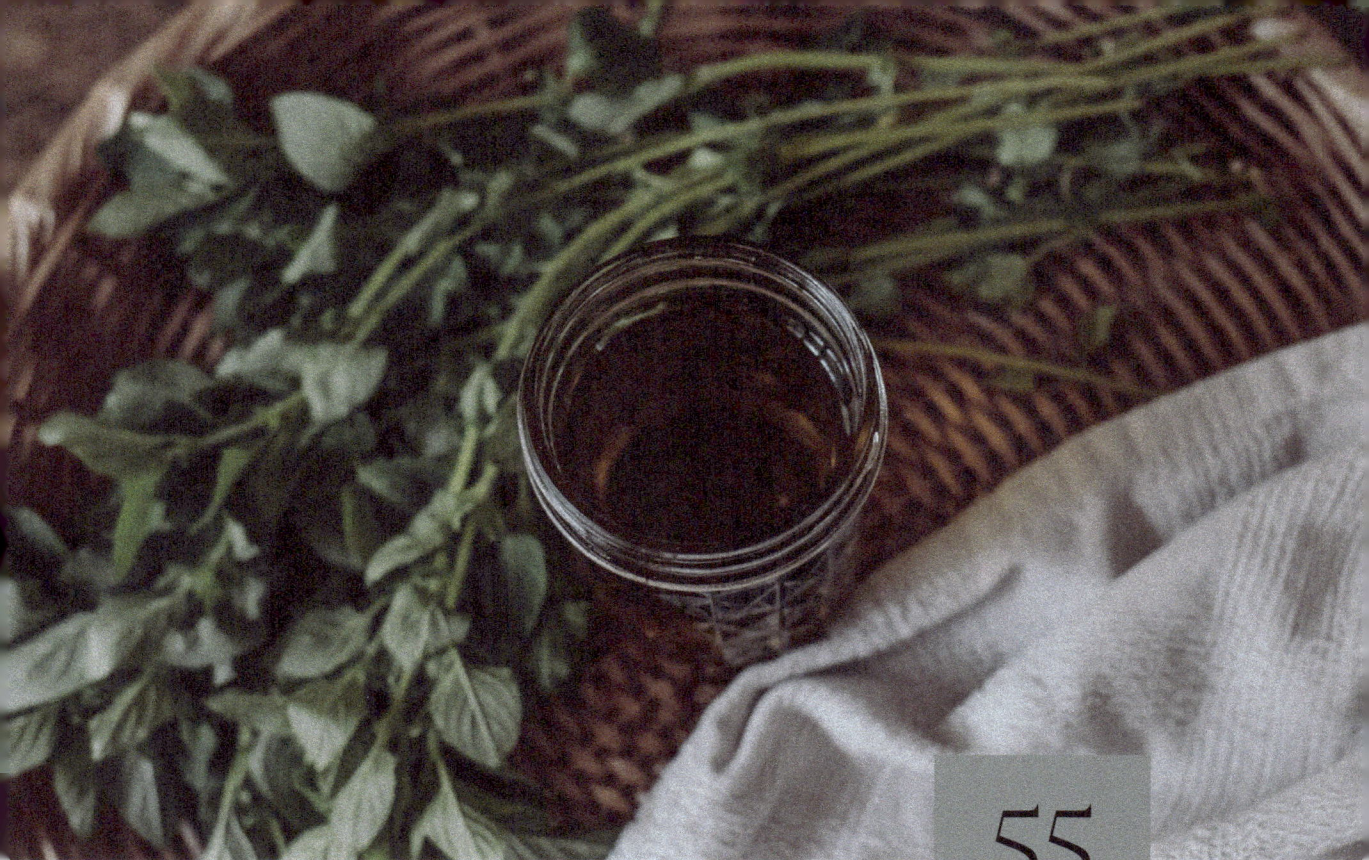

Oil of Oregano

Oil of oregano is a traditional herbal remedy going back possibly thousands of years and has been used for everything from ear infections to digestive upset. Oregano is anti-microbial, anthelmintic (destroys parasites), analgesic, as well as antioxidant, making oregano an extremely versatile and useful herb.

The method of extraction for this particular oil utilizes fresh oregano in order to preserve as much of its volatile oil as possible. When using fresh herbs in oils, its important to keep an eye out for mold or rancidity. Any time moisture is introduced to oil, such as with fresh herbs, it opens up the opportunity for mold to develop or the oil to degrade.

Large bunch fresh oregano sprigs
1/2 cup high quality extra virgin olive oil

Rinse oregano and dry thoroughly. Strip leaves from stems, and roughly chop. Place chopped leaves in the upper bowl of a double boiler, bringing water below to a low simmer.

Add oil and stir to combine. Cover and let warm for 1-5 hours. Use a thermometer to be sure the temperature remains between 100-105 degrees.

Remove from heat and strain. Store in a well-sealed jar in a cool dark place. Use as needed.

Strain 4 Thieves Vinegar

The 4 thieves vinegar that you made on day 28 has been macerating for over 4 weeks. It is now ready to be strained. Remember, if any mold is visible, or a rancid smell emanates from the jar – dispose of the vinegar and start over.

To strain: line a fine mesh sieve with cheesecloth over a large bowl. Pour the infused alcohol and herbs over the cloth. Use the cloth to wring out any alcohol remaining in the herbs. Dispose of herbs and cheesecloth.

Once strained, store the tincture in a sealable dark glass jar or bottle. Place jar in a cool dark spot for up to one year.

Uses:

Immune boostin – take 1 Tbsp 1-3 times daily when you feel a cold coming on, or someone else in the house is ill.

Cleaning – place undiluted 4 thieves vinegar into a spray bottle and use directly on a surface. If the surface is greasy, add a small amount of water and castile soap. Be careful, as the acid content of the vinegar can deteriorate some surfaces. Be sure to check how to care for the surface before use.

Vinaigrette – blend together 3 Tbsp extra virgin olive oil, 1 Tbsp 4 thieves vinegar, pinch of salt, and 1 tsp of Dijon mustard.

Bug Repellent – place in a spray bottle that is partially diluted with distilled water. Spray as necessary on the body.

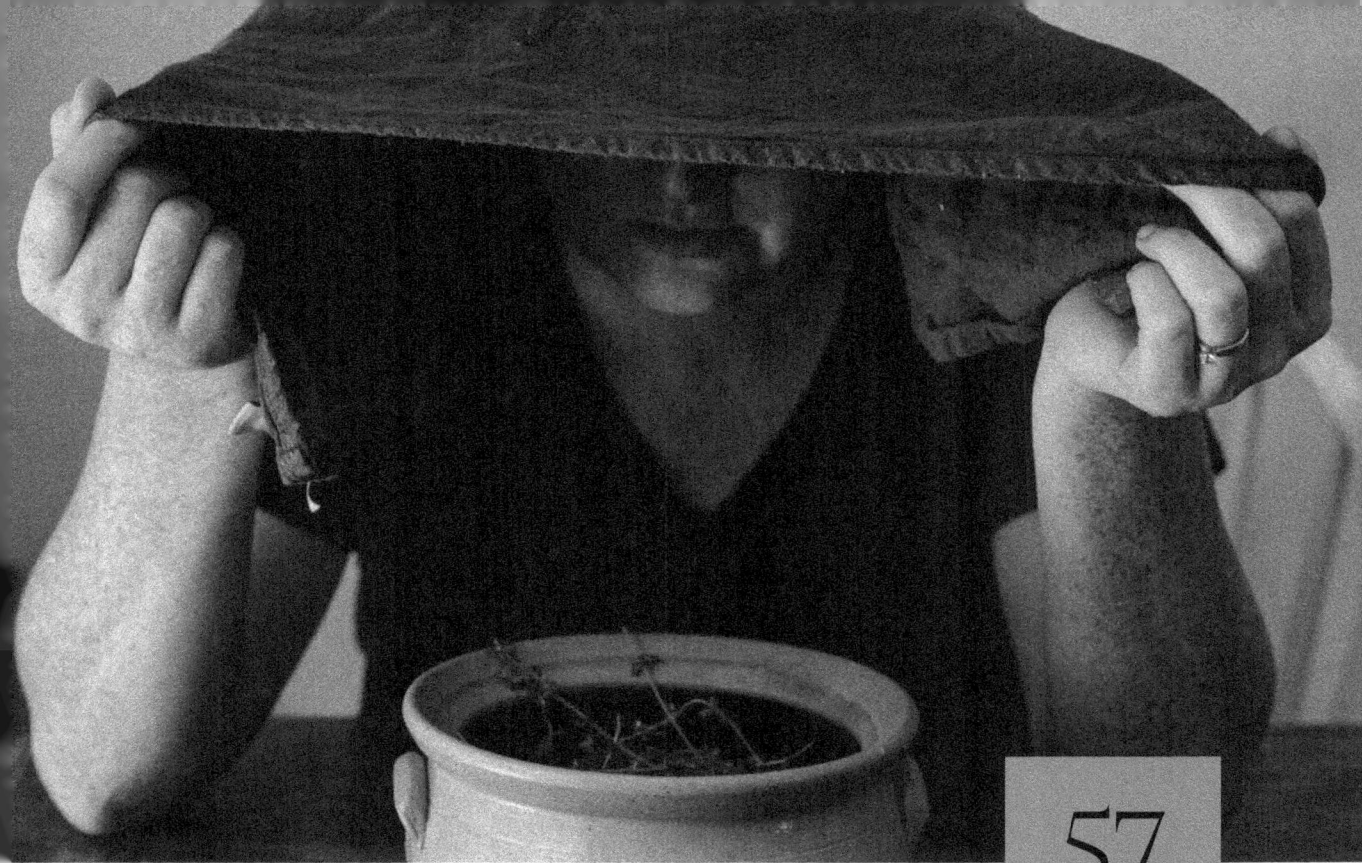

Herbal Steam for Sinuses

Steam is a fabulous method for reducing mucus congestion. Adding herbs can increase the effectiveness of the steam, while providing additional benefits depending on the herbs selected.

1 cup water boiling water
2-3 Tbsp herbs

Place herbs in a large mug and pour boiling water over top. Position head over bowl, with closed eyes, and drape a towel over to create a tent to hold steam.

Inhale deeply though the nose and remain tented for 5-10 minutes.

Repeat throughout the day as needed.

Refer to day 17 to find herbal actions that can help with sinus congestion. Some good herbs for sinus steams:

Oregano - expectorant, anti-microbial

Thyme - expectorant, anti-microbial

Rosemary - relieves stagnant congestion in sinuses and lungs

Mullein leaf - relaxes lungs, alleviates dry cough

Eucalyptus - loosens mucus

Chamomile - relieves cough, Inflammation

Yarrow - reduces swelling, dries excess mucus

Clove - expectorant, anti-microbial

First-Aid Tincture

This first-aid tincture utilizes the anti-microbial power of alcohol, along with the wound healing capabilities of herbs like yarrow, thyme, and lavender. It is a key component to any home apothecary and is used topically to help disinfect cuts, scrapes, and mild burns.

0.5 oz yarrow (by weight)
0.3 oz thyme (by weight)
0.2 oz lavender (by weight)
5 oz 120 proof vodka (by volume)

Combine herbs and alcohol in a sterile mason jar. If alcohol does not cover the herb, you will need to add more. Be sure to measure and record the additional amount.

Line the lid with unbleached paper and screw on tightly. Label with ingredients, measurements, and date.

Place jar in a dark area. Allow mixture to infuse for 4-6 weeks, shaking occasionally.

Turn to day 93 for straining and use instructions.

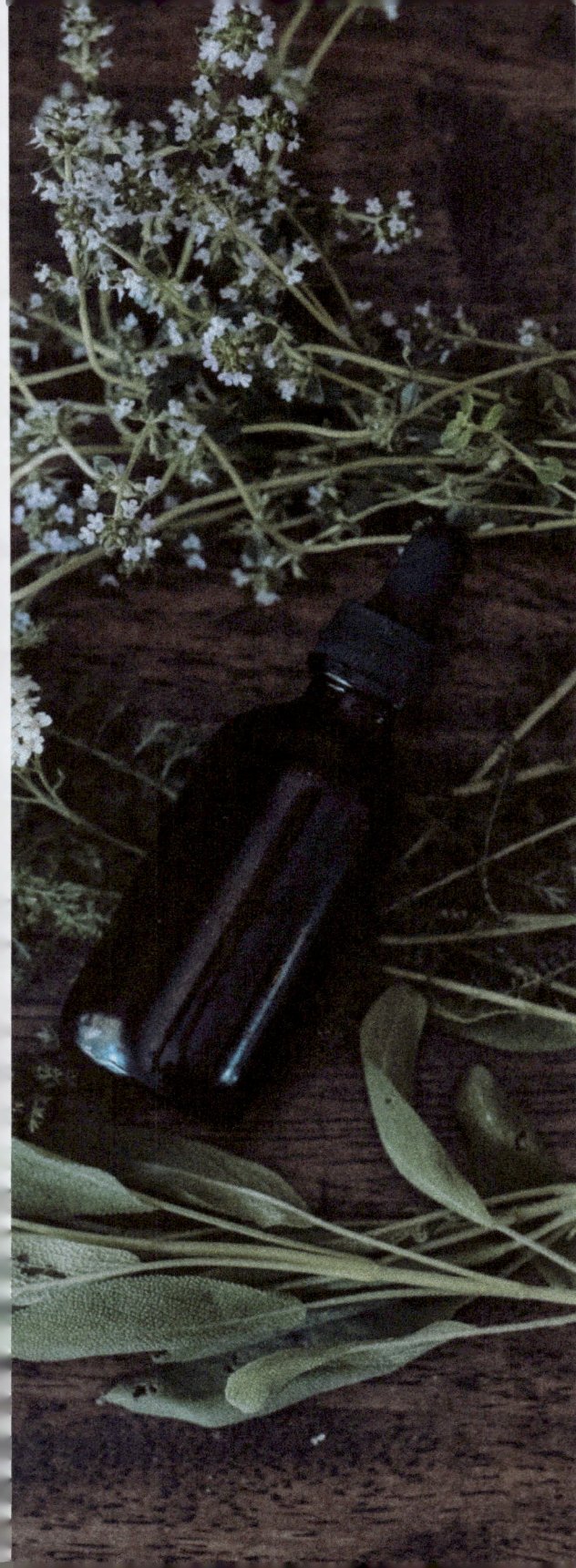

Cold Sore Lip Balm

Lemon balm (Melissa officinalis) is a powerful anti-viral herb that has been shown to work against the herpes strain of viruses that cause cold sores. Utilizing a lip balm infused with lemon balm can reduce the occurrence and severity of cold sores.

In addition to its anti-viral power, lemon balm is bitter, diaphoretic, anti-spasmodic, nervine, carminative, antidepressant, antioxidant, and radio protective. It's many benefits and low maintenance tendencies make it an exceptional plant to grow in the garden and keep on hand. Unfortunately, it has been shown to interfere with the function of the thyroid for those with thyroid issues.

Salve Instructions

1/2 cup lemon balm heat infused oil
2 Tbsp beeswax
1 drop vitamin E
10 drops tea tree essential oil (optional)

Combine infused oil and wax in the top of a double boiler. Fill the bottom of the double boiler with 2-3 inches of water, bringing to a light simmer to gently heat oil and wax.

Continue to heat and stir occasionally, until all wax has dissolved. Be sure to heat until there are no ripples in the surface of the oil; this means that the wax is fully dissolved.

Remove from heat and stir in vitamin E and essential oils.

Carefully pour mixture into jars or tins to cool. Once cooled, a solid ointment should remain.

To use: Rub fingers across the surface of the salve to pick up a small amount and apply to the affected area as desired.

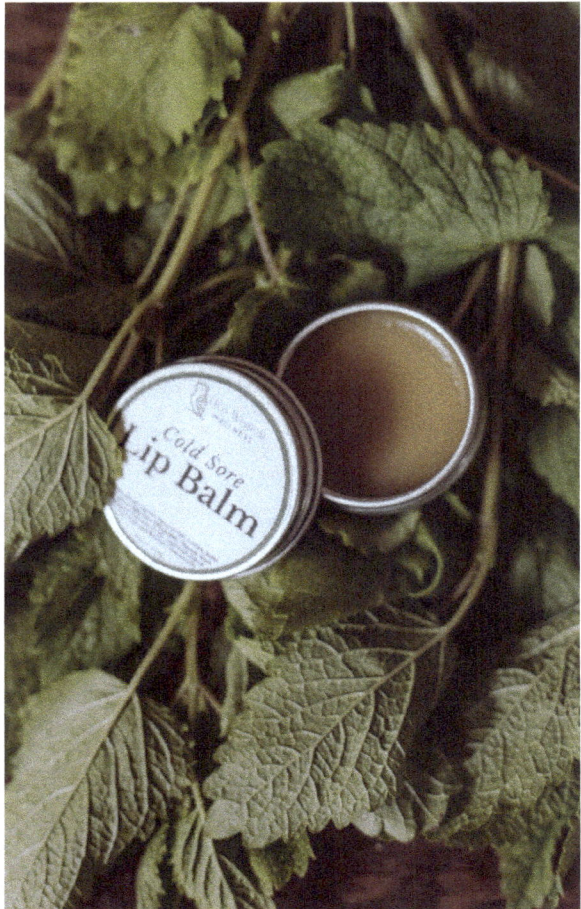

Dandelion Chicory Coffee

Both chicory and dandelion have wonderful earthy, coffee-like tastes, especially when roasted. This combination is often used as a non-caffeinated alternative to coffee that is both delicious and contains amazing health benefits.

Dandelion (Taraxacum officinalis) is a liver tonic known to support digestion, excretion, to balance blood sugar, and more.

Chicory (Chichorium intybus) shares many of the same benefits as dandelion root, and is also a kidney tonic.

For this recipe, it is recommended to purchase roasted root powders. However, if that is not possible, opt for roasted roots and powder them by the same method described on day 27. If you cannot obtain roasted roots, you can purchase dried roots, roasting them the same way you would roast coffee beans.

Dandelion Chicory Coffee

2 cups water
1 1/2 Tbsp roasted chicory root powder
1 tsp roasted dandelion root powder
Milk of choice (optional)
Sweetener (optional)

Bring water to a boil and pour over chicory and dandelion. Steep for 10-20 minutes.

Strain with a coffee filter or french press.

Pour into mugs, adding milk and/or sweetener as desired.

Serve warm.

Iced Coffee Version:
Increase chicory root powder to 2 Tbsp and the dandelion root powder to 1 1/2 tsp

Once steeped and strained, pour warm liquid over ice, adding milk and/or sweetener as desired.

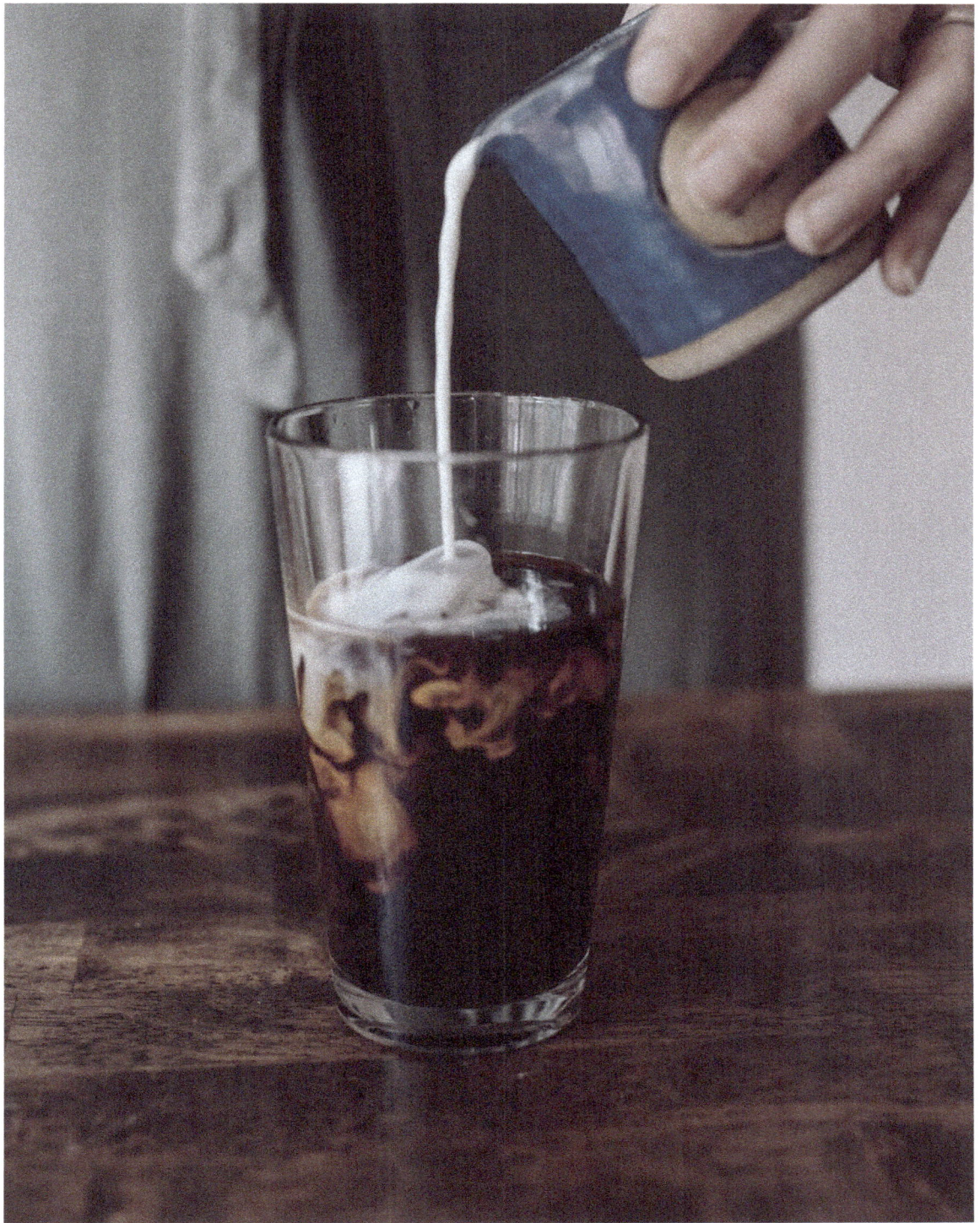

Rosemary's Famous Face Cream

This recipe, direct from famous herbalist Rosemary Gladstar, creates a thick and luxurious face cream that is deeply moisturizing and healing. While calendula is an incredible herb for skincare, feel free to add or change herbs based on your skin type. Herbs like rosemary, lavender, chamomile, rose, or yarrow are great options. Go back to day 26 for more information on herbs for skin care and day 12 for more information on choosing oils to use.

3/4 cup calendula infused oil
(equal parts grapeseed and apricot or oil of choice)
2 Tbsp cocoa butter
2 Tbsp coconut oil
1 rounded Tbsp beeswax pastilles
1/4 cup commercially prepared aloe vera gel
3/4 cup distilled water
10 drops lavender essential oil

Combine infused oil, cocoa butter, coconut oil, and beeswax in a double boiler until fully melted and well blended.

Remove from heat and let cool at room temperature overnight. The mixture should become mostly firm, but soft in the middle.

Scrape the cooled oil/butter mixture into a blender.

In a separate bowl, whisk together aloe vera, water, and essential oil.

Turn on the blender and slowly drizzle in water mixture. The mixture should emulsify to become thick and creamy.

Store in well sealed jars, in a cool dark place for up to a year.

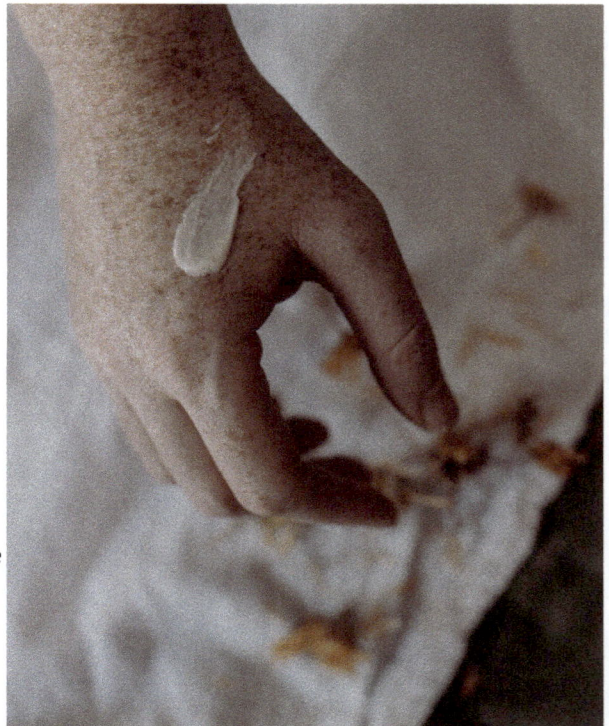

Foot Baths

Herbal foot baths are an overlooked health practice that have multiple benefits. The feet are one of the hardest working parts of our body, and hold a lot of our stress and tension Supporting them regularly can not only help them stay strong and supple, but also reduce stress and tension. Foot baths are known to increase circulation, nerve function, prevent clotting, and to reduce foot odor and fungus.

Basic Foot Bath
1 gallon hot water
1/4 cup herbs
2 Tbsp Epsom salt
additional add-ins as desired

Allow water to cool enough to put your feet in. Let sit for 20-40 minutes. Ideally, you want to start sweating slightly before removing your feet. This indicates that circulation has begun.

If using additional liquid add ins, reduce amount of water accordingly.

Anti-Fungal
4-5 cups apple cider vinegar
clove
cinnamon
ginger

Sore Foot
4 Tbsp baking soda
peppermint
wintergreen leaves
chamomile

Goddess
1/2 cup powdered milk
fresh lemon slices
rose
lavender
chamomile

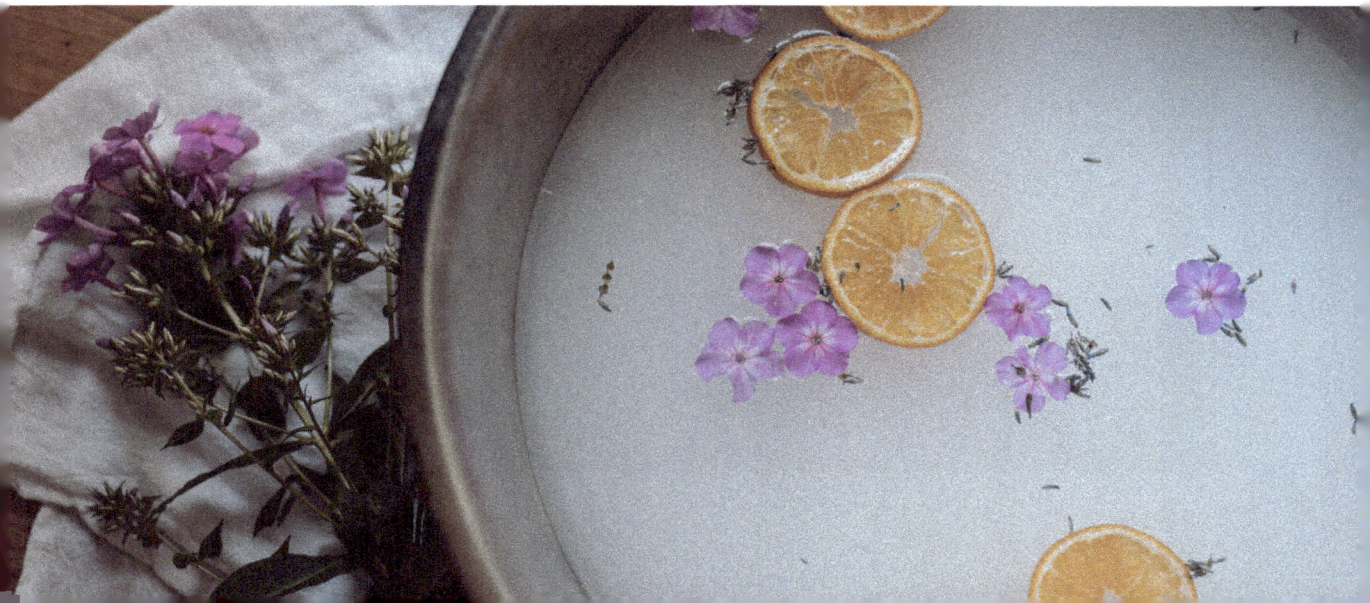

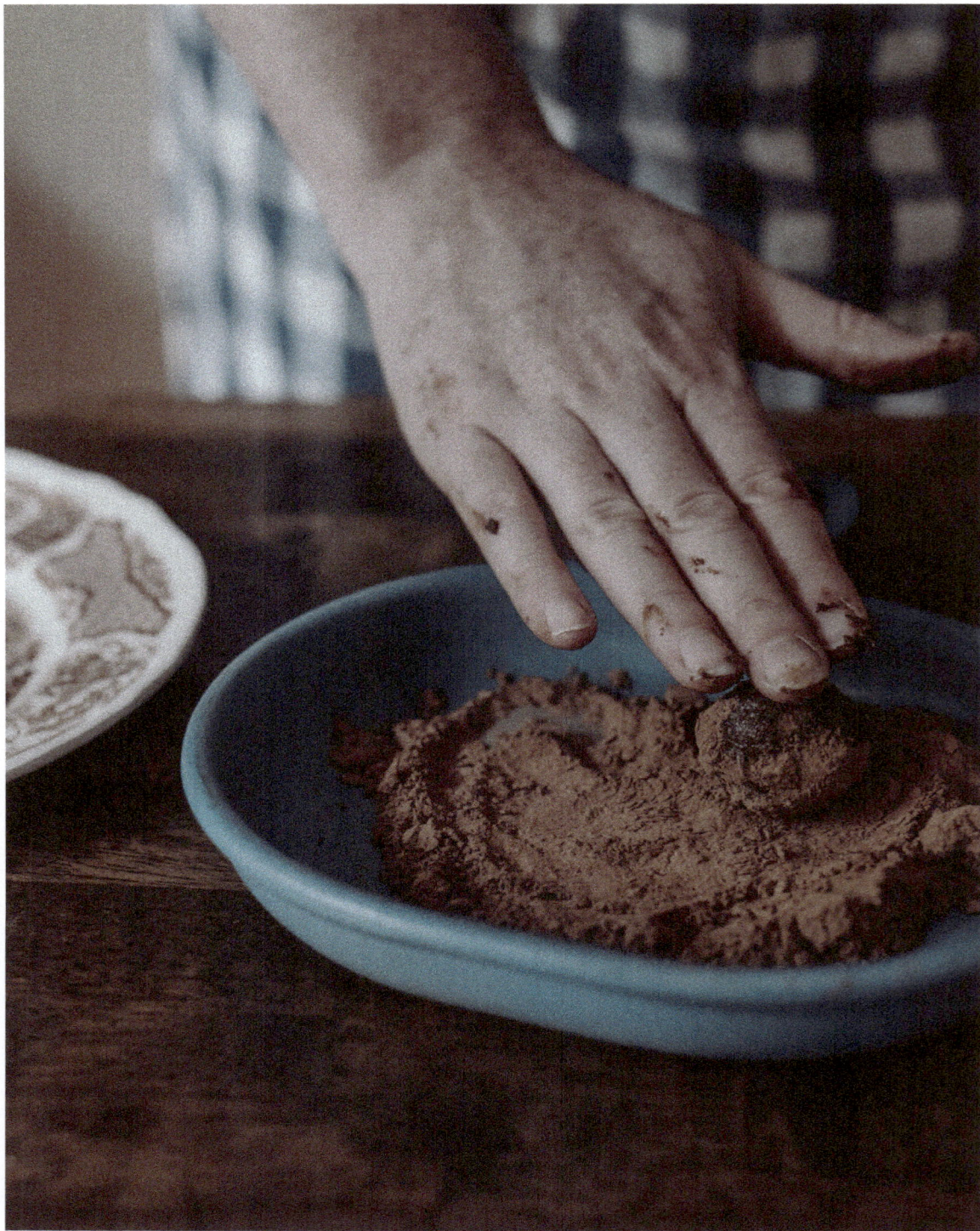

Adaptogen Power Balls

In times of stress, regular use of adaptogens can be helpful to balance the adrenal system, helping the body respond to the symptoms of stress. Incorporating adaptogens in delicious and indulgent ways, such as power balls or protein cookies, are great for supporting your body with high quality foods.

15 dates, pitted
½ cup cashews
½ cup walnuts
1 Tbsp water
1 Tbsp reishi mushroom powder
1 Tbsp ashwagandha powder
½ cup raw cacao powder
2 Tbsp honey
Toppings (toasted coconut, cacao powder, powdered sugar, etc.)

Combine dates and cashews in a large bowl. Cover with water, and let sit for 10-15 mins.

Drain, then blend together dates and cashews with walnuts in a blender until combined.

Add water, reishi powder, cacao, and honey. Continue blending until smooth, scraping down the sides of the blender as necessary.

Place in fridge for 30 minutes to 1 hour to firm up.

Scoop out mixture and roll into 2 inch balls (a rounded tablespoon volume).

Roll balls in your topping of choice, and serve.

Store in fridge for up to 1 week.

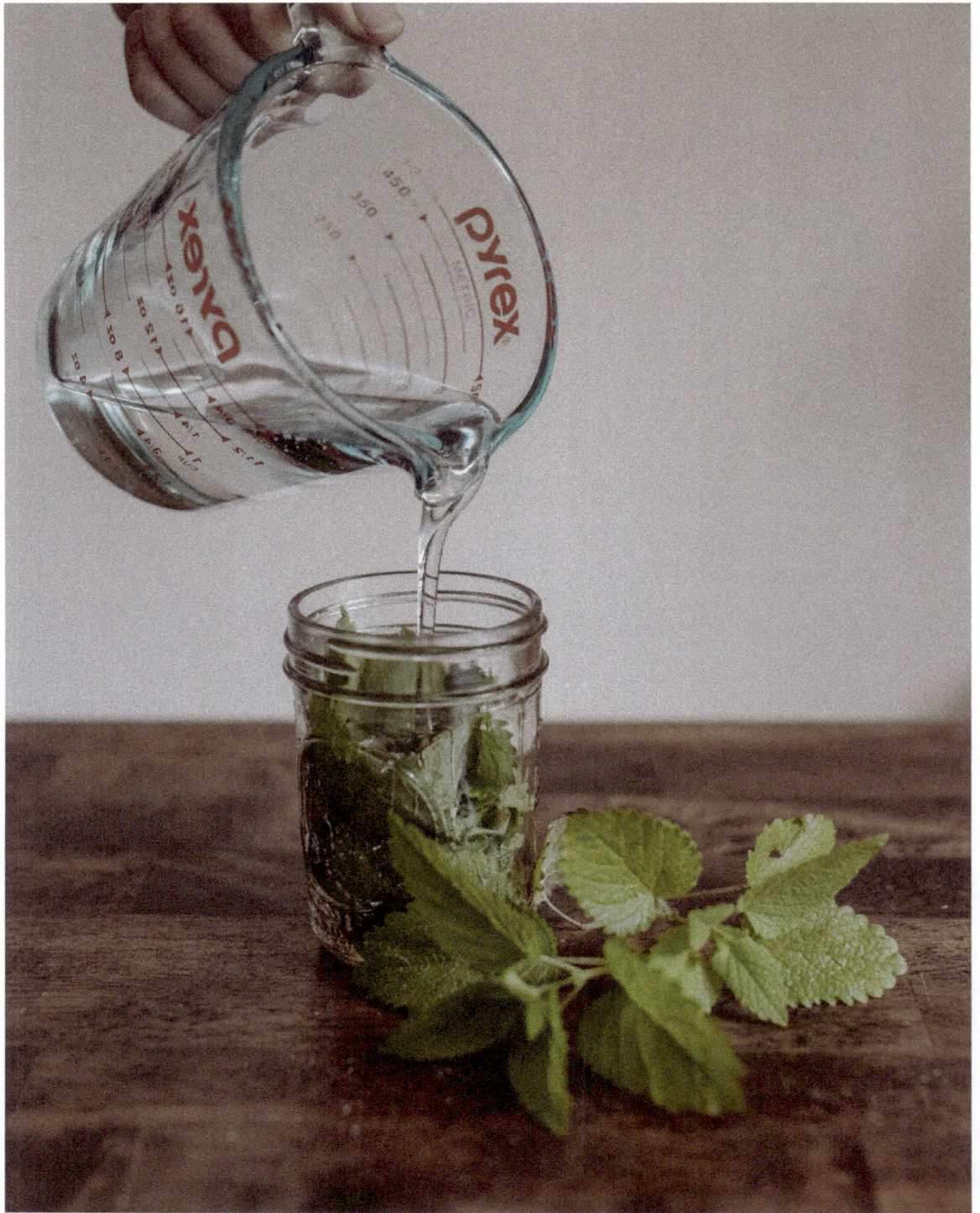

Lemon Balm Glycerite

A glycerite is a potent liquid herbal extract made with glycerin. It is similar to a tincture, except that it is non-alcoholic. A glycerite is typically a clear, odorless liquid with a syrup-like consistency. While it is sweet in flavor, it is not metabolized like sugar. This makes it an optimal choice for small children, those avoiding alcohol, and for those with blood sugar issues.

Look for an organic, sustainably harvested, non-GMO glycerin to use in medicine-making. It is important to note that glycerin is not as effective in extracting compounds from dried herb matter as an alcohol tincture would be, so it will be slightly less potent. Just like alcohol extracts, an herbal glycerite dosage can vary greatly depending on the plant. Most recommendations for glycerites are double the dose that would be recommended for an alcohol tincture of the same plant. For example: a tincture of lemon balm (1:5 45% alcohol) typically has a dosage of 2-6ml up to 3 times daily, making the glycerite dosage 4-12 ml (or 1-2 tsp) up to 3 times daily.

Lemon Balm Glycerite

Fill a sterile jar with chopped fresh plant material or half-full of dried plant material.

For fresh plants, add enough glycerin to fully cover the plant matter, filling the jar while leaving 1 inch of room on top. If using dried herb, dilute glycerin with distilled water in a 3:1 (glycerin:water) ratio. Fill jar with mixture, leaving 1 inch of room on top.

Use the end of a clean wooden spoon to gently press herb under the glycerin to ensure the release of air bubbles, allowing maximum coverage of materials. Cover with a tight fitting lid, and give a gentle shake to distribute.

Let sit for 4-6 weeks, shaking every 1-2 days. Be sure the plant matter stays below the surface of the glycerin. If it continues to float, use a sterile weight to keep it below the surface (a sterilized rock works nicely).

Strain and store in a glass bottle in a cool dark place.

A well-stored glycerite will have a shelf life of 1-2 years.

For additional uses and ideas, turn to day 94.

65

Herbs for Pain & Inflammation

White Willow Bark - (Salix alba) White willow bark has been used for centuries, typically in the form of tincture or tea, to reduce pain and inflammation. The salicin compound found in white willow bark was used to develop the main ingredient in modern day aspirin. It is often employed to help with headaches, muscle pain, inflammation, joint pain, and osteoarthritis.

Devils Claw - (Harpagophytum procumbens) Despite originating in southern Africa, Devil's claw has been widely used in Europe for hundreds of years. It is used for the treatment of arthritis, headaches, and low back pain, but it can help with general pain and inflammation. This herb tends to have a harsh taste, and is often used in tincture form.

Ginger - (Zingiber officinale) As one of the planet's most popular herbs, ginger has been used both internally and externally for generations in Asian, Indian, and Arabic cultures. Ginger is used for issues associated with inflammation and pain. The anti-inflammatory compounds in ginger function in a similar manner as COX-2 inhibitor drugs (such as ibuprofin or tylenol), that are also used to treat pain and inflammation.

Arnica - (Arnica montana) When used topically, arnica has been shown to help reduce soreness, bruising, swelling, and pain associated with minor injuries.

Yarrow - (Achillea millefolium) Known for it's role in the myth of Achilles, yarrow has been used for centuries for a multitude of wound-healing purposes. It has shown benefits for everything from pain associated with IBS and period cramps, to wound healing and mouth sores.

Comfrey - (Symphytum officinale) Also called knit bone for its ability to generate new cell growth and promote wound healing, comfrey is also useful topically for pain, inflammation, bruising, and sprains.

Cayenne - (Capsicum frutescens) The same constituent, capsacin, that makes these peppers spicy is also responsible for its ability to block the transfer of pain signals to the brain, therefore relieving pain. It can be used both topically and internally for this use.

Rosehip - (Rosa spp.) In addition to containing constituents that have been known to help reduce joint inflammation and damage, rose hip has been shown to help relieve general lower back pain as well. Rosehip is typically used internally, as a tincture or a tea.

Peppermint - (Mentha × piperita) Peppermint is known to help physically relax muscles, easing soreness and tension. It is often employed topically for head and neck tension, headaches, and back pain. Internally, it can help with gastric upset and heartburn.

Bruise/Sprain Compress

Sprains, strains, and bruises can cause a lot of pain and annoyance. Utilizing healing herbs both topically and internally can quickly ease some of the symptoms of these types of injuries.

Most of us are familiar with the acronym RICE for Rest, Ice, Compression, and Elevation; however, recent studies have shown that this method can actually be detrimental to the healing process with these types of injuries. Instead, it is suggested to continue movement as long as it doesn't hurt too much, and avoid using ice or compression which can impede blood flow to the area. Heat can be applied after the initial surge of swelling has reduced, in which case, feel free to use a warm compress. To start with, keep the compress at a fairly neutral temperature, as too much heat initially can increase swelling.

1 part dried comfrey leaf
1 part dried arnica
1 part dried yarrow

Combine all herbs together, using 1 Tbsp of herbs for every 8 oz of water to create a strong infusion. When cooled, dip a cloth into the infusion, squeezing out excess water. Place on injured surface and let sit 5-10 minutes. Remove for 10-20 minutes. Repeat 2-3 times, as needed.

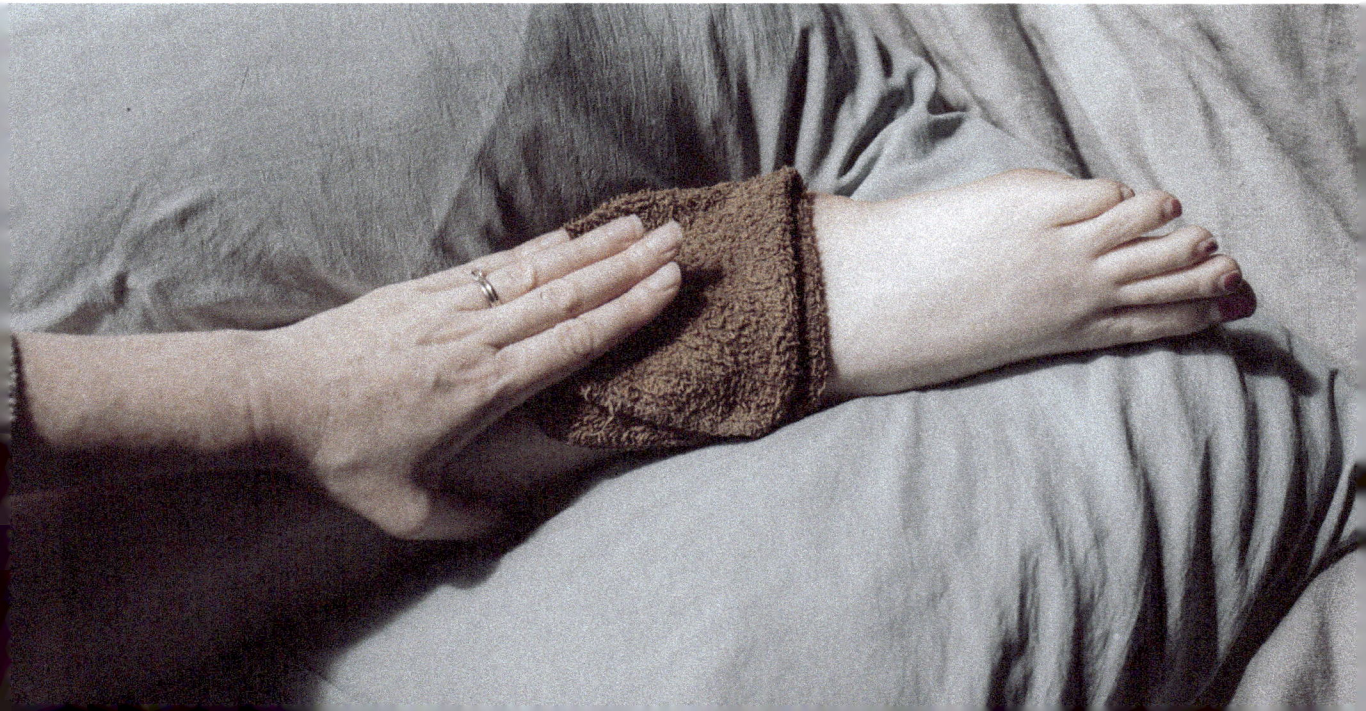

Make Fire Cider

Another modern classic, created by Rosemary Gladstar; Fire Cider has been used by thousands of herbalists over several decades. It utilizes a number of spicy, pungent, immune-boosting herbs, giving it a fiery flavor and the source of it's name. This particular recipe uses the addition of raw honey to help mellow out the flavor and make it more palatable.

Classic Fire Cider

6 cloves garlic
1/4 cup ginger, sliced
1/4 cup turmeric root, sliced
1 Tbsp fresh oregano sprigs
1 Tbsp fresh thyme
peel of 1 lemon
2 cayenne peppers
1 1/2 cups raw apple cider vinegar
3 Tbsp raw honey

Combine herbs in a pint jar and pour vinegar over top. Add honey and seal tightly.

Invert several times to ensure contents are well coated, and the honey and vinegar are mixed.

Set it in a cool dark place for 4-6 weeks. Be sure to give the jar a good shake regularly, keeping contents well coated.

After 4-6 weeks, strain well and discard herbs.

Store in a sealed container for 4-6 months, using as desired.

Use 1 Tbsp up to 3 times daily during times of cold and flu.

Turn to day 91 for additional information on decanting and uses.

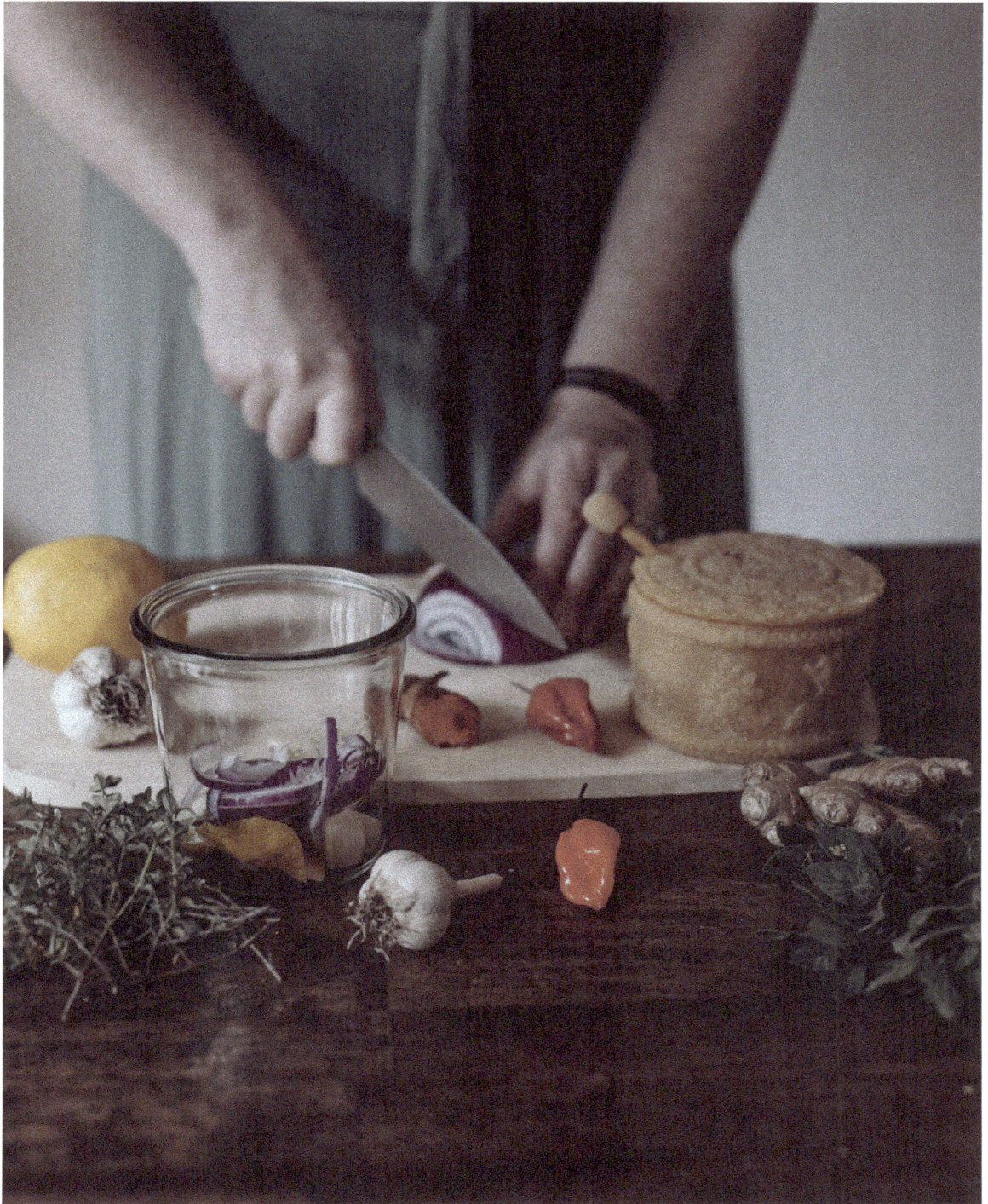

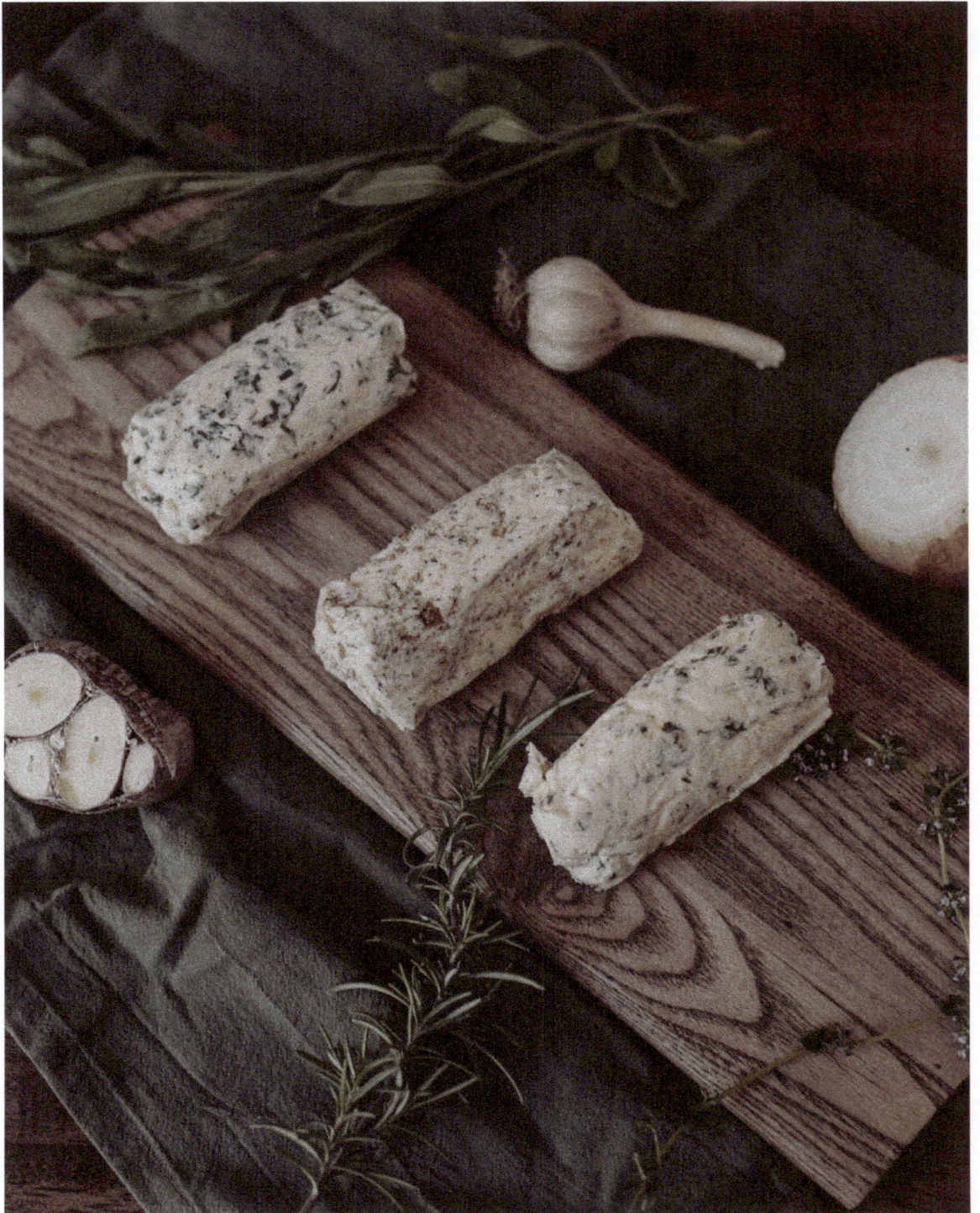

Compound Butter

Compound butter is one of the most versatile ways to incorporate herbs on a regular basis, as well as in times of need. They can be made ahead and stored in the freezer until needed, or whipped up in a few minutes with both fresh and dried herbs.

Serve them as part of a meal, or on a slice of bread to administer medicine. Few people will say "no" to bread and butter – even when they are battling an upset stomach! They also make delicious host gifts around the holidays, or when traveling.

Basic Compound Butter Recipe

2-3 Tbsp fresh herbs
1 stick (4 oz) butter, softened
1 tsp sea salt

Place softened butter in a bowl with herbs and salt. Use a fork to mash and blend completely. Use as desired.

To shape: transfer butter to a square of wax paper. Use the wax paper to roll butter into a log shape. If the butter starts to melt, place in the fridge to solidify for 5-10 minutes. Once shaped, use or store in the fridge for up to 1 week or the freezer for several weeks.

Immune Blend

1 Tbsp crushed garlic
1 Tbsp minced oregano
1 tsp minced sage
1 tsp minced thyme

Lung Support

1 Tbsp minced plantain leaf
1 Tbsp minced sage
1 Tbsp minced oregano

Stress Relief Blend

1 Tbsp minced tulsi
2 Tbsp minced lemon balm
1 tsp grated lemon peel

Digestive Warmer

1 Tbsp ground cinnamon
1 Tbsp shredded ginger
1 tsp ground clove

69

Styptic Powder

Styptic powder is an antiseptic clotting agent that stops bleeding by contracting the blood vessels. It is very beneficial to have on hand for things like cuts on the head, nose bleeds, or paper cuts.

To make this treatment, simply dry and powder constricting herbs like yarrow. To powder, combine the herbs in a clean coffee grinder and pulse. Once they are mostly powdered, sift them through a fine sieve to remove any large pieces that could abrade the skin. Sprinkle a small amount of the powder directly on the wound (or inside the nostril) to slow bleeding.

Yarrow (Achillea millefolium) - Often called the warrior plant, yarrow derives its scientific name from an old Greek legend. The legend of Achilles tells how Achilles' mother dipped him into a pool of yarrow tea, to protect him from harm. He grew to become a valiant warrior and was only vanquished by a wound to the ankle – the only place that the yarrow infusion had not reached.

Mostly known for it's antiseptic, anti-inflammatory, and astringent properties, yarrow has a long history of being used to help heal wounds, bruises, and sprains on the battlefield, naturalizing across the globe as it traveled with numerous armies over thousands of years.

Note: Yarrow is not safe for use with pets.

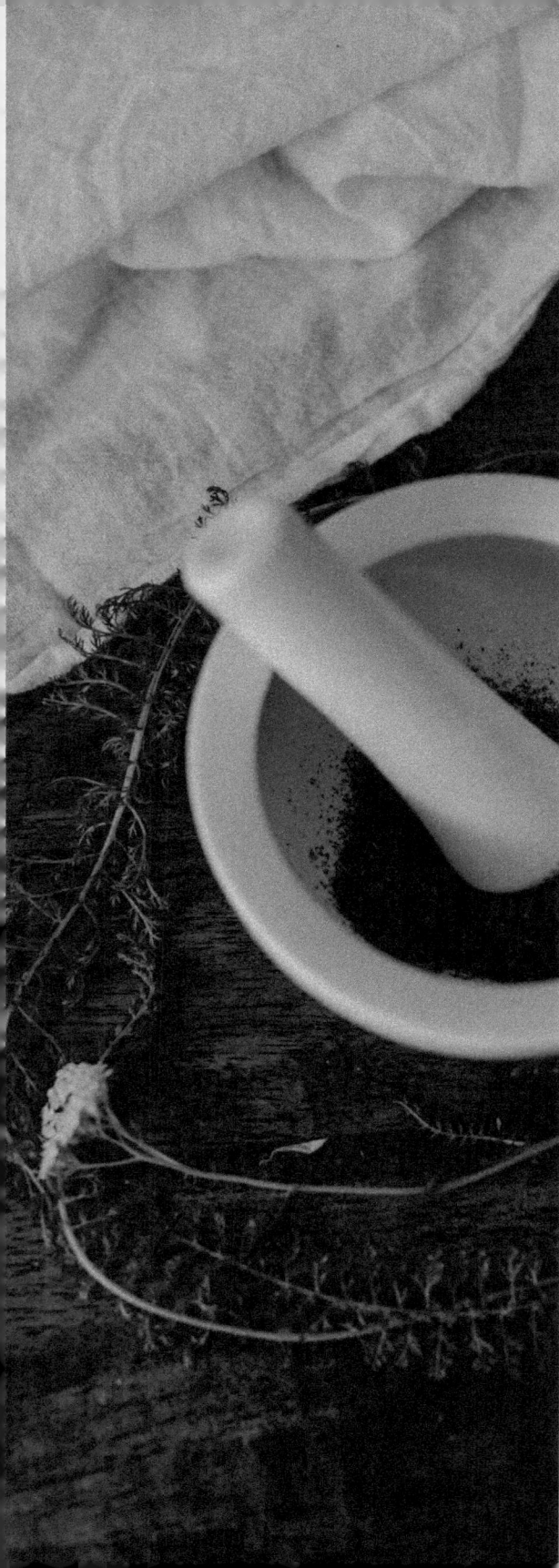

Cayenne Bone & Joint Rub

Cayenne is a very hot and spicy herb due to the constituent capsaicin. It is also responsible for the herb's pain relieving power. Capsaicin reduces a substance in humans that is used to send pain signals to the brain, providing relief for things like arthritis, joint pain, back aches, and bruises.

Salve Instructions

1/2 cup oil of choice
2 tsp cayenne powder
2 Tbsp beeswax
10 drops ginger essential oil (optional)

Combine cayenne powder and oil in a mason jar or in the bowl of a double boiler.

Gently heat herbs over very low heat (90° and 120° F) for 3-5 hours.

Remove from heat and allow to cool slightly.

Strain liquid with a cheese cloth lined mesh strainer. Several layers of cheese cloth with be needed, as the powder is fine.

Combine infused oil and wax in the top of a double boiler. Fill the bottom of the double boiler with 2-3 inches of water. Bring to a light simmer to gently heat the oil and wax.

Continue to heat, stirring occasionally, until all wax has dissolved. Be sure to heat until there are no ripples in the surface of the oil; this means that the wax is fully dissolved.

Remove from heat. Stir in essential oils, if using. Carefully pour mixture into jars or tins to cool. Once cooled, a solid ointment should remain.

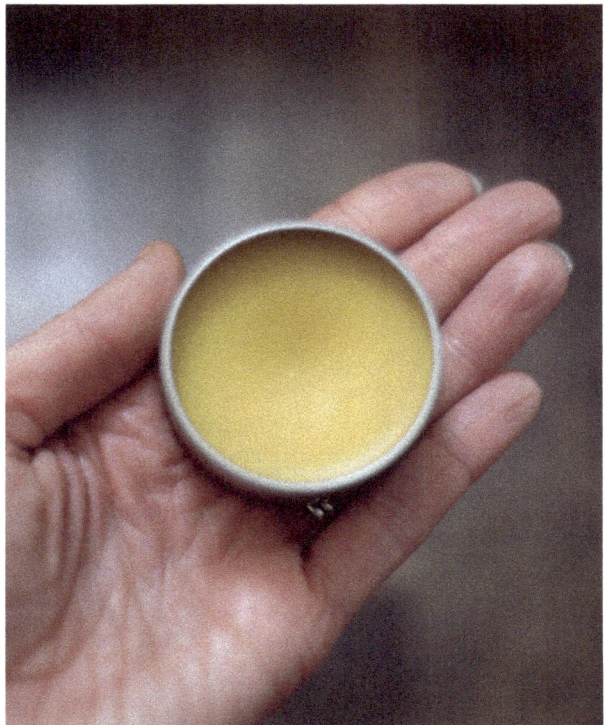

Raspberry Electrolyte Popsicles

Homemade popsicles are a great and tasty way to make sure everyone in the family is stays hydrated on hot summer days, especially kids. They can be made even more nourishing by adding mineral and antioxidant-rich herbal teas. The sweetness of fresh fruit and syrup makes even bitter herbs delicious for youngsters.

Popsicles are a great way to help alleviate the symptoms of a sore throat. For this purpose, try soothing herbs like chamomile, licorice, mallow, ginger, or peppermint.

Raspberry Electrolyte Popsicles
1/2 Tbsp raspberry leaf
1/2 Tbsp nettle leaf
1/2 Tbsp hibiscus
2-6 Tbsp maple syrup
handful fresh raspberries, crushed
juice from 1 lemon
pinch baking soda

Combine the raspberry leaf, nettle, and hibiscus in a quart sized, heat-safe jar. Pour boiling water over top. Let steep for 10-20 minutes.

Strain and stir in maple syrup to taste, crushed raspberries, lemon juice, and baking soda until well blended. Pour into molds. Freeze thoroughly and enjoy.

Turmeric Moon Milk

In traditional Ayurvedic medicine, steamed milk was used as a vehicle for administering medicines, such as turmeric and ashwagandha. This concept has been popularized in modern times as milk lattes, or moon milks.

This recipe focuses on the benefits of turmeric and ginger, with supporting herbs such as such as cinnamon, cardamom, and black pepper. Together, this blend is highly anti-inflammatory and antioxidant, as well as supportive of digestion and circulation.

1/4 inch piece fresh ginger
1 1/4 tsp ground turmeric
3-4 cardamom pods
1/3 tsp ground cinnamon
pinch black pepper
1/4 cup water
1 cup milk of choice
1/4 tsp vanilla extract
1-1 1/2 Tbsp sugar

In a small sauce pan combine ginger, turmeric, cardamom, cinnamon, pepper, and water.

Bring to a simmer, and let cook for 3-4 minutes.

Reduce heat to medium. Pour in milk, vanilla, and sugar. Mix well and heat until milk begins to steam. Do not let boil. As soon as steam begins to appear, remove from heat.

Strain into a mug, use a milk frother if desired. Serve hot.

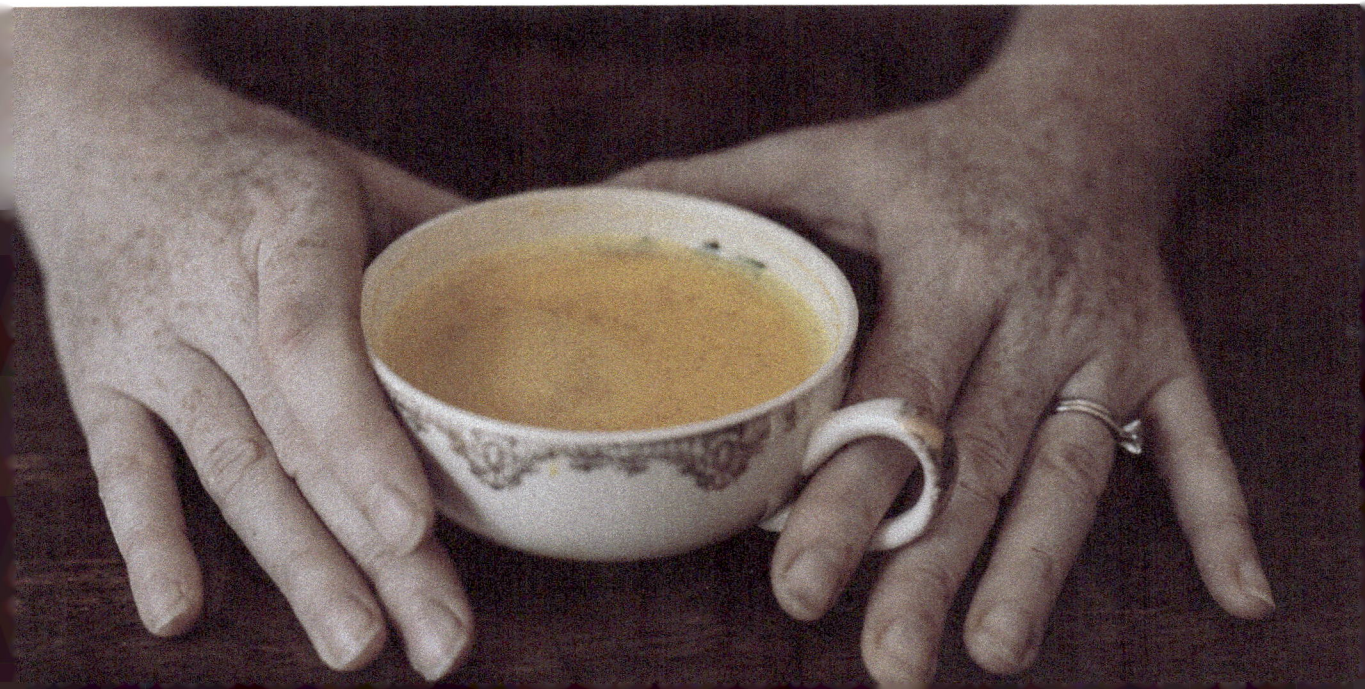

Learn Botany Basics

Botany is the study of plants, and is an important topic for herbalists of all levels. Not only is it necessary to identify plants correctly, but to identify plant families and their corresponding characteristics. Most herbal botany is focused on naming and classification for this reason.

Classifications

Classifications are used to help identify organisms. Classification begins with Kingdoms and are broken into 5 parts: Animalia (animals), Plantea (most plants), Fungi (mushrooms & lichen), Prositsa (some algae and flagellates), and Monera (cyanobacteria, and some algae). Next Phylum, Class, and Order further break down these categories into smaller groups. Typically, for the study of herbalism, the focus remains on the final three classifications of an organism. Those being family, genus, and species.

Family - Organisms in the same family are so alike that they will have similar structures and constituents, and therefore will usually have similar actions.

Genus - Usually the first word in the scientific name of a plant. Many organisms in the same genus are similar enough to have the ability to interbreed.

Species - The most specific unit of classification. This distinguishes variations in genus, some specifics may include varying colors of specific plant genus.

Chamomile

Kingdom - Plantea (plant)
Phylum - Tracheoppyta (vascular plants)
Class - Magnoliopsida-dicotyledons
(flowering plants with paired leaves)
Order - Asterales (flowers with densely aggregated stamens)
Family - Asteraceae (heads composed of many small florets, surrounded by bracts)
Genius - Matricaria
Species - Chamomilla

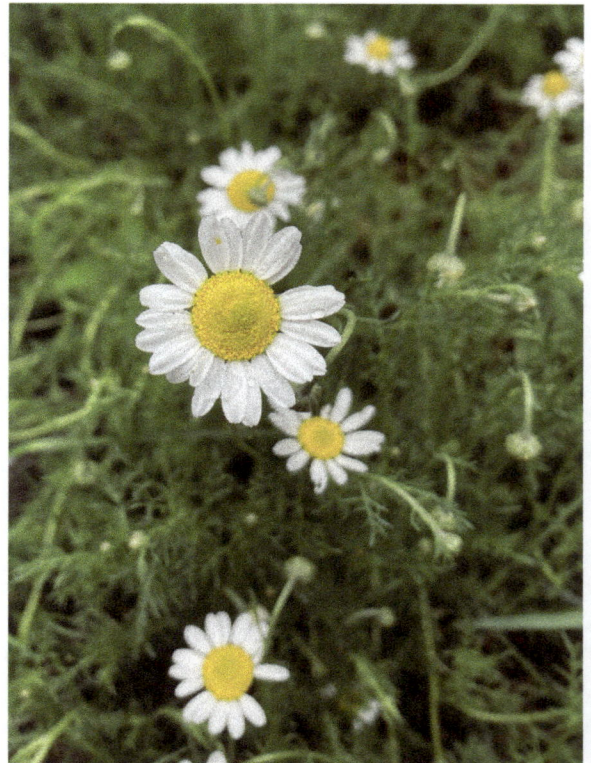

Botany Basics Activity

Pick a few plants and identify their catagories. How are they similar or different? Do you notice any commonalities in certain catagories?

Plant Common Name   Plant Common Name

Kingdom   Kingdom

Phylum   Phylum

Class   Class

Order   Order

Family   Family

Genus   Genus

Species   Species

Plant Common Name   Plant Common Name

Kingdom   Kingdom

Phylum   Phylum

Class   Class

Order   Order

Family   Family

Genus   Genus

Species   Species

Understanding Plant Parts

Plants have many parts that all have different types of tissues, cells, and functions. It is important to understand the different parts of a plant, as they can each have different constituents and actions. On some plants, the root could be medicinal while the leaf or fruit can cause unpleasant symptoms. This is an important distinction to make when working with plants. Use a botany reference book to identify different parts of the plant.

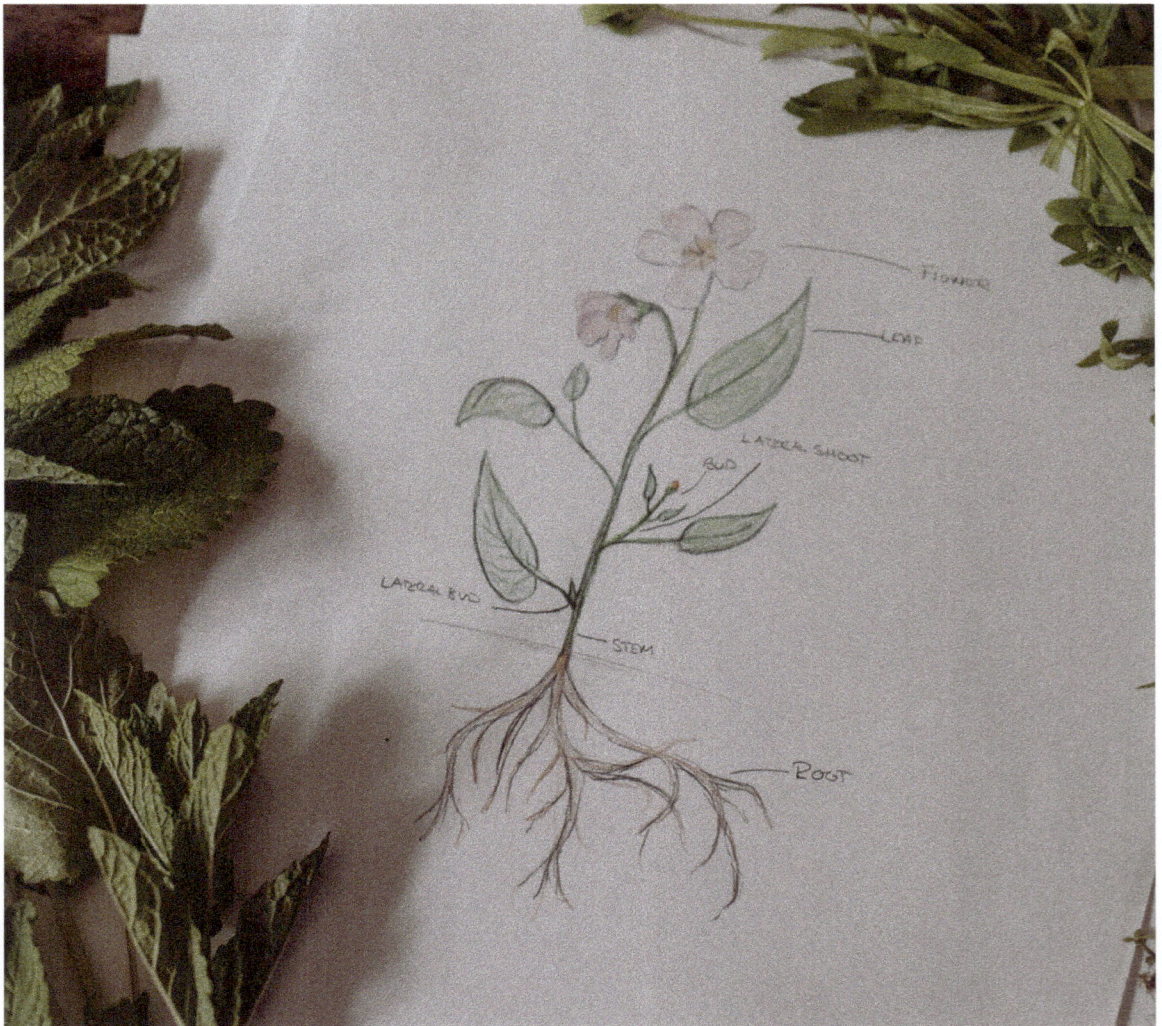

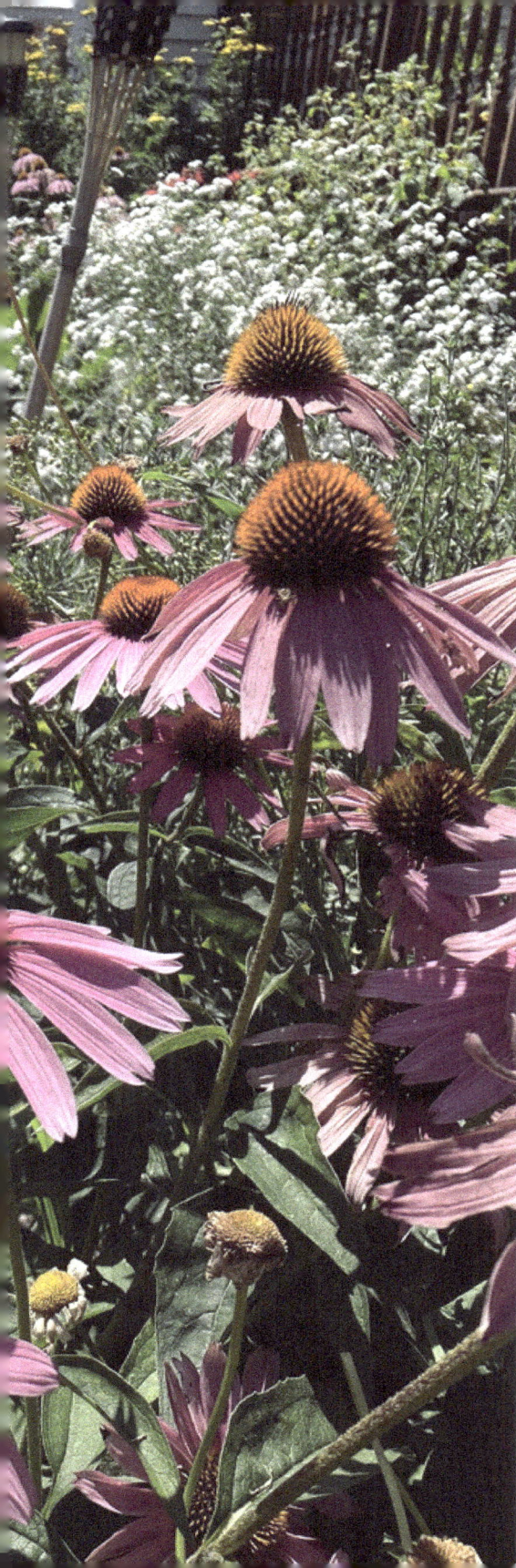

Go for a Plant Walk

Use this walk as an opportunity to try and find similarities in the plants that you can identify. Write them down or take photos. Take some time to research them. Find out which ones are in the same families and what actions they may have.

Mints

Mint has many members in its family (lamiaceae); including familiar herbs like lemon balm, catnip, basil, and oregano. Members of this family are easily identified by their square stems and oblong leaves that are often serrated. They usually have narrow tips and range in color from dark to light green.

Daisies

The Asteraceae, or daisy, is another broad family that encompasses a large number of plants including echinacea, calendula, and dandelion. These family members can be identified by their flower, which while appearing to be a single flower with larger "ray petals around the outside" are actually made up of many tiny disk flowers at it's center.

Mustards

The mustard (Brassicacaea) family includes well known vegetables such as broccoli, cauliflower, and cabbage. The wild plants in this family can be identified by their mustardy or peppery odor and flavor. The flowers tend to be small, with four cross-shaped petals. Plants in this family are often used for digestive issues, respiratory irritation, and as food.

76

Draw a Plant

Choose one of the plants from your plant walk to draw. Identify it's different parts and any distinguishing features that helped you to identify it.

Sage Salt Gargle

Gargles are used to relieve a sore throat, and can also be used regularly to help support the lymph and immune systems prior to getting sick. The action of gargling helps to reduce inflammation and sinus congestion in acute situations. It helps to relieve allergies, colds, sore throats, and respiratory infections.

Adding herbs like sage to a gargle can help enhance these benefits. Sage is antiseptic, anti-inflammatory, nervine, and antispasmodic; helping to relieve sore throats, cough, and infection, as well as helping the body and muscles of the throat relax.

Sage Salt Garlge

1 cup boiling water
1 Tbsp dried sage
pinch salt

Pour hot water over sage and salt.

Cover and let stand for 10-15 minutes.

Strain and use to gargle as needed.

Can be made ahead and kept in the fridge for up to 1 week.

Warm gently prior to use.

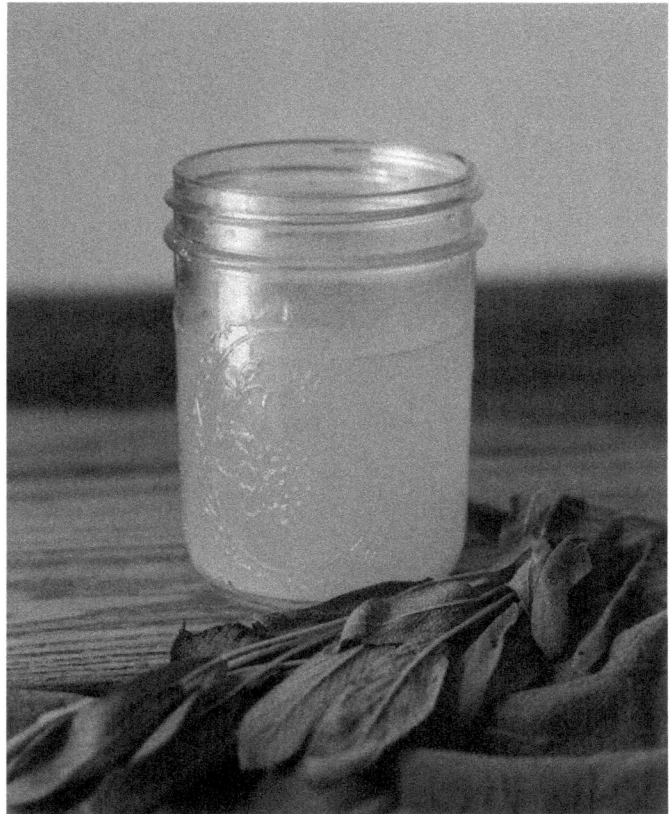

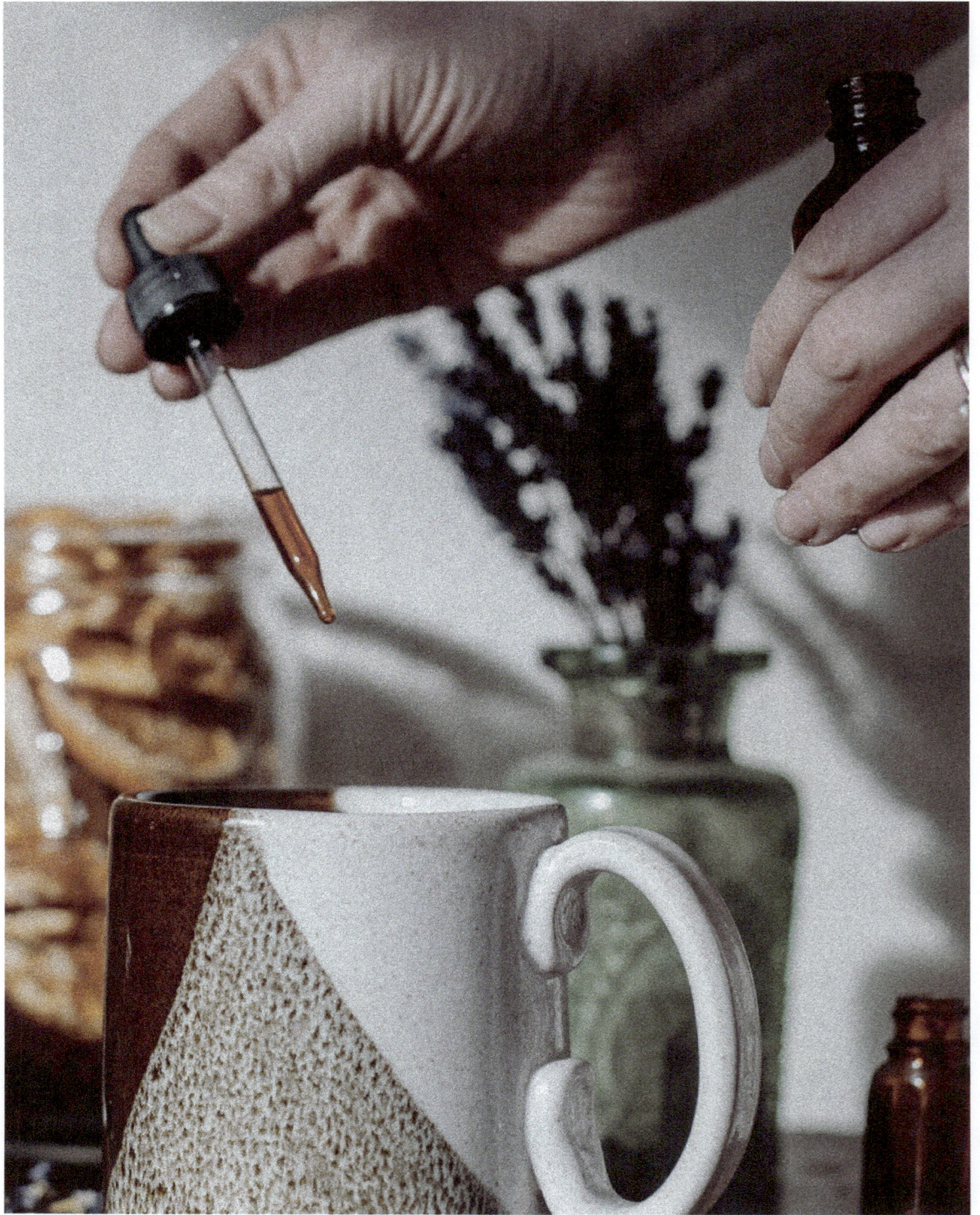

Strain Ashwagandha Tincture

The Ashwagandha tincture made on day 32 has been macerating (soaking or infusing) for over 6 weeks, which means it is time to strain it. Tinctures can remain unstrained without much spoilage, but the safest way to ensure that mold or rancidity does not occur is to strain and store properly.

Line a fine mesh sieve with cheesecloth over a large bowl. Pour the infused alcohol and herbs through the cloth. Use the cloth to squeeze out any remaining alcohol from the herbs. Dispose of or compost the herbs and cheesecloth.

Once strained, store tincture in a sealed, dark glass jar or bottle. Set in a cool dark place for up to one year.

Dosage: 1-3 ml of tincture taken 1-3 times daily.

How to Use Tinctures

Typically, tinctures are stored in dropper bottles. The droppers administer about 1-2 ml each use.

A dropper-full can be taken directly under the tongue (be sure not to touch the dropper with your mouth to avoid contaminating it with bacteria). Other popular ways to take tinctures are by adding a dropper-full into a shot glass of water, or adding it to another drink.

More on Ashwagandha

(Withania somnifera) is native to Southeast Asia and Africa. It has been used for thousands of years in Ayurvedic medicine and in some West Asian cultures. Its name (ashwagandha) loosely translates to the strength and smell of a horse in the sacred Hindu language of Sanskrit. This eloquently describes not only the smell of the plant, but its ability to boost stamina, energy, and strength. Studies have shown that regular use of the herb can help improve the stress response and anxiety for some. It has been shown to improve athletic performance, balance blood sugar, and support sex hormone production in some men. Historically, asgwagandha has been used throughout Southern Asia for immune system support, adrenal fatigue, thyroid support, and even as an aphrodisiac.

Create a Sore Throat Blend

Teas are often one of the first lines of defense against a sore throat, and luckily there is a herb for just about every cause of a sore throat there is.

When creating a blend for a sore throat, it's important to think about the cause of the issue. Is it instigated by a post nasal drip? Does the mucus need to be dried up or moved out? Herbs like peppermint, sage, and thyme can be beneficial for this kind of instance. Is the coughing the result of an irritating respiratory issue? Perhaps a lung tonic like mullein, along with soothing anti-spasmodic or democulent herbs would be a great combination.

Take note of the type of sore throat you are addressing, and create a blend for it. Use the space below for notes as needed.

Oat Bath for Skincare

Oatmeal baths have long been used as home remedies for numerous skin ailments including rash, eczema, chicken pox, and dermatitis. Oats are emollient, meaning they soften and soothe tissues they come in contact with. This makes them a perfect option for a soothing bath.

Typically, the oats are ground into a fine powder in a coffee grinder or high powered food processor. This not only increases surface area of the herb, but allows it to release it's medicinal components more easily into the water. Additionally, it stops the oats from clogging the tub drain.

Additional herbs that can be added to soothe and repair skin include lavender, calendula, and chamomile.

1 cup powdered oats
1/4 cup powdered herbs

Combine ingredients in a warm bath and soak for 15-20 minutes. Gently towel dry skin and apply moisturizer as desired.

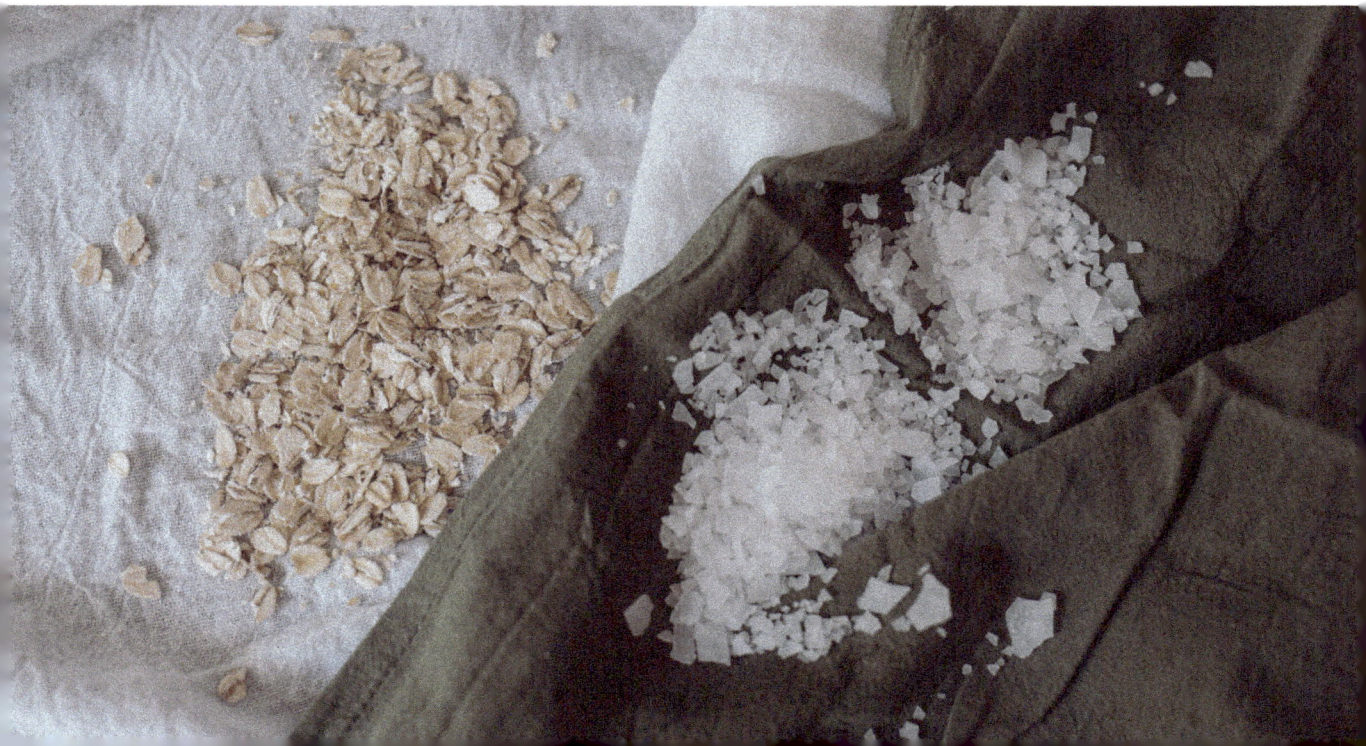

Headache Compress

The benefits of using an herbal compress for headache relief are multi-fold. The scent of many herbs can trigger reactions that alleviate headaches, but their constituents can also be absorbed through the skin to provide relief as well.

Placing a warm compress on the head and face or neck can allow the herbs to work directly on the affected areas providing faster relief.

Herbs like mint and lavender can help relieve tension in muscles, which lead to tension headaches. Herbs like chamomile work to reduce inflammation and eye strain.

Headache Blend

1 part peppermint
1 part spearmint
1 part yarrow

Eye Strain Blend

2 parts chamomile
1 part fennel
1 part lavender
1 part yarrow

Combine all ingredients in a tea strainer to brew a strong cup of tea.

Make sure tea has cooled enough to avoid burning the skin. Dip cloth into the warm tea and wring slightly so it is not dripping.

Place cloth on the skin and let sit for 5-10 minutes.

Repeat as necessary.

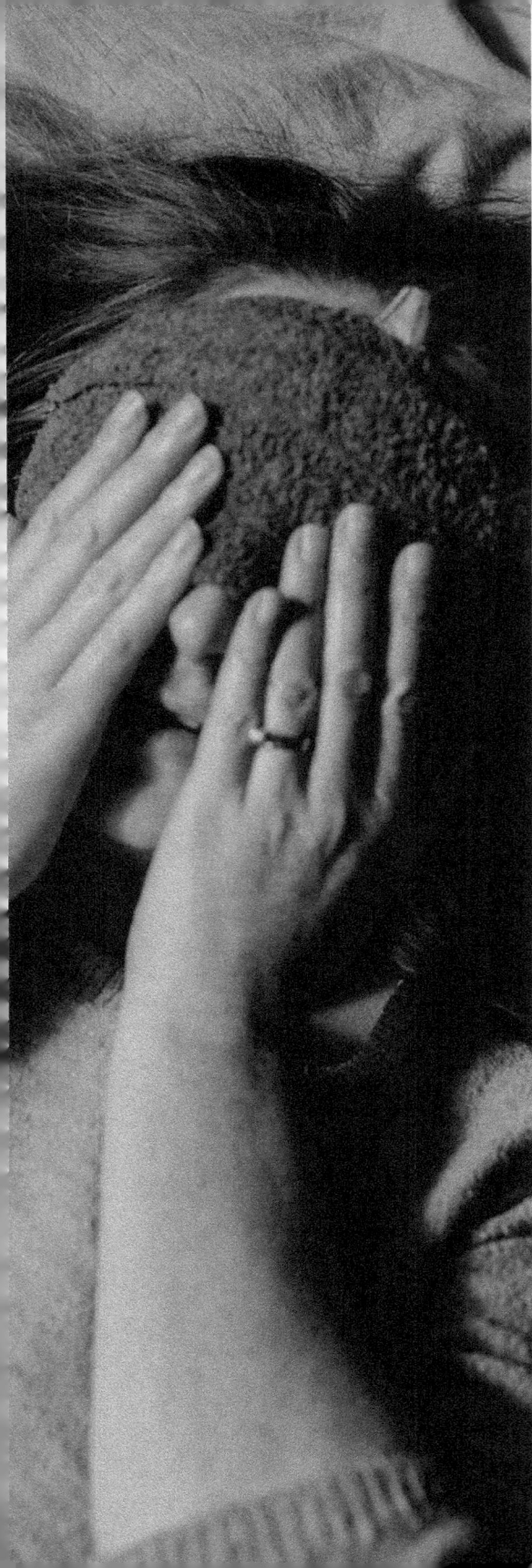

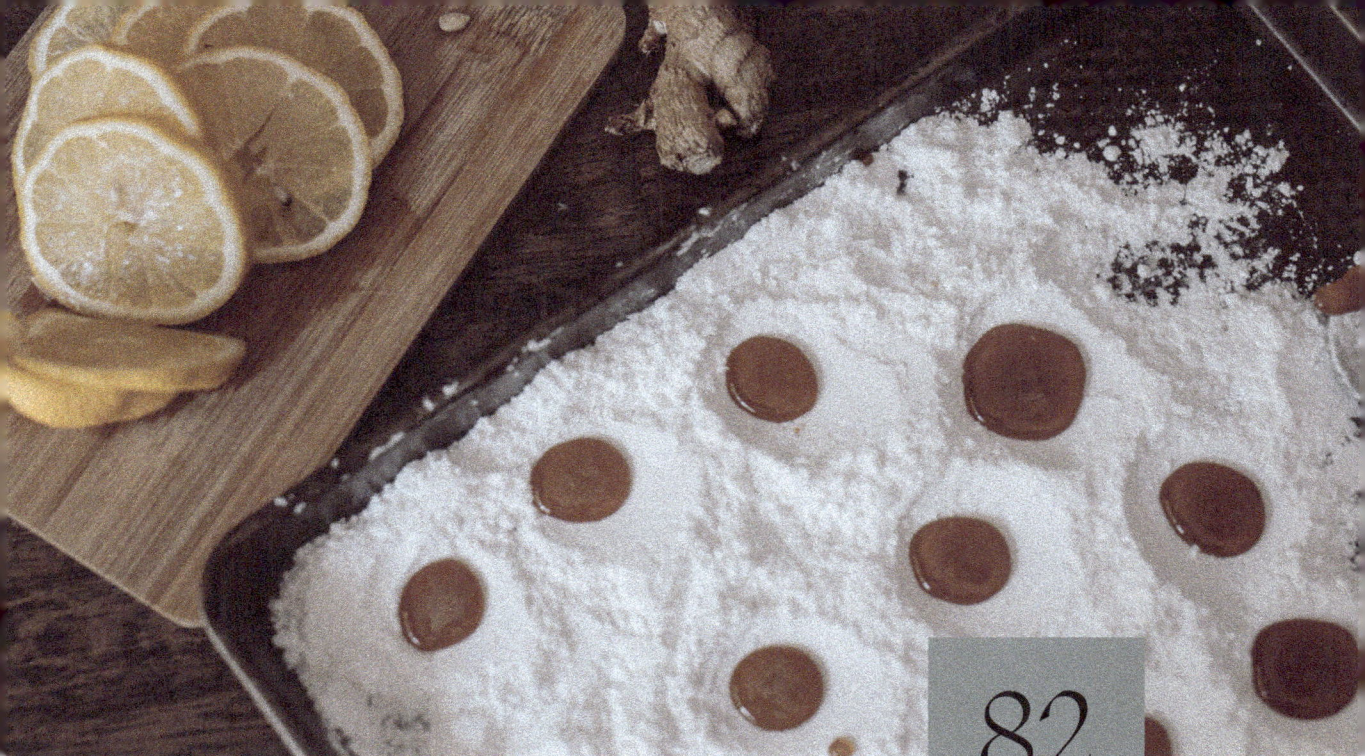

Lemon Ginger Cough Drops

½ cup honey
2 Tbsp fresh lemon juice
1 tsp fresh grated ginger
Powdered sugar, for coating

Combine all ingredients in a thick–bottomed saucepan over medium-low heat. Stir regularly to keep mixture from scorching.

Continue to cook until mixture becomes bubbly and foamy. Turn down heat slightly, continuing to cook. Use a candy thermometer to heat mixture to be between 300-310F. If you don't have a candy thermometer, you can drop some of the mixture into a bowl of ice water. If it hardens into a candy, then it is at the correct temperature.

Once mixture has reached this hard candy stage, remove from heat and allow it a couple of minutes to cool and slightly thicken.

Pour mixture into candy molds, or a plate covered with 1 inch of powdered sugar. Allow to cool until hard and firm. Dust with powdered sugar to prevent the candies from sticking.

Store in a sealed container in a cool dry place.

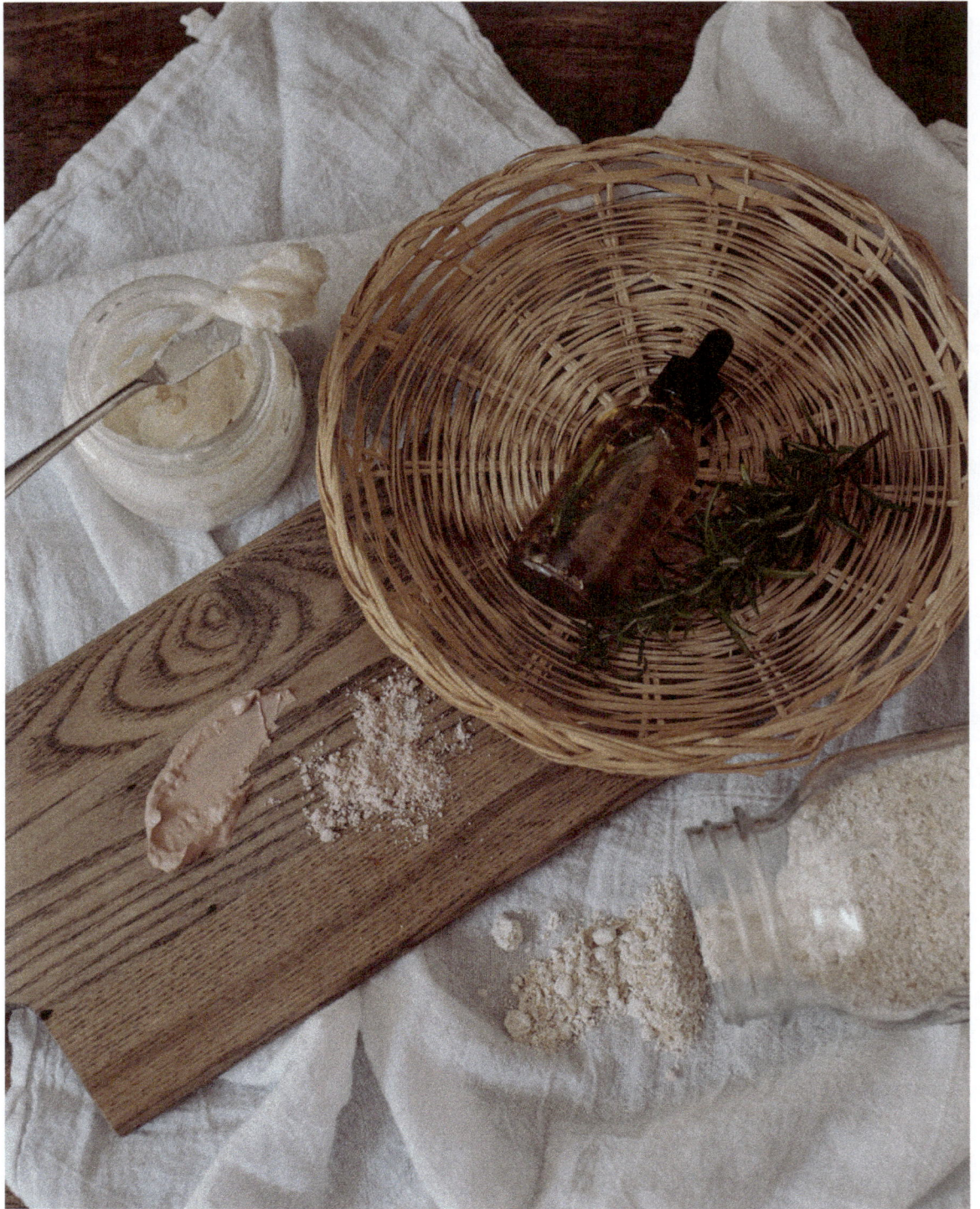

Herbal at Home Facial

At-home facials are a great way to practice self-care while also protecting your skin from the effects of daily exposure. Below are the steps for a typical facial. Use the skills you've gained and recipes you've already made throughout your 100-day journey to create your own customized experience. The entire at home facial process may take several days to complete, if you do not already have these items on hand. Simply go through, and choose the ingredients and recipes you would use for yourself and your specific skin type.

1 Cleanse - Combine 3 Tbsp castile soap, 2 Tbsp water, and 1 Tbsp infused oil, such as the calendula oil created on day 23, the blend from day 13, or create a new one based on your skin type with the information provided on day 12.

2 Exfoliate - Use finely powdered herbs or baking soda with an herbal infused oil (like the above) to form a paste. Gently massage into skin, then wash off by splashing warm water on your face.

3 Steam - Turn back to day 37 to find information on creating your own herbal face steam.

4 Clay Mask - Create a custom mask with the recipes and herbs discussed on day 26 and 27.

5 Tone - There are many options for toners; you can use plain witch hazel or rose water (day 44), or use a tea made from astringent herbs like rosemary, sage, or chamomile.

6 Hydrate - Serums will add hydrating, skin balancing, repairing, or anti-aging elements to your skin. Use the oil infusing method from day 13 or day 23 to make a serum.

7 Moisturize - Moisturizers are a must and can be as easy or as complicated as you like. A simple salve (days 24) with skin-loving herbs is one option, or try a whipped herbal blend (day 53), or Rosemary's famous face cream (day 61).

Fermented Onions

Onions are for more than just cooking. They are known for their anti-bacterial, anti-oxidant, and anti-diabetic qualities. Onions are used to boost the immune system, and to support healthy gut bacteria. The following fermented onion recipe includes additional spices that can aid digestion and immune support. Turn to day 90 for uses and recipes.

Fermented Onions

1 lb red onions, thinly sliced
1 1/2 Tbsp kosher salt
1/2 cup water
1 tsp spices (cumin, coriander, black pepper, fenugreek, mustard)

In a large mixing bowl, combine sliced onions, and salt. With your hands, massage onions until they are coated in salt and begin to sweat.

In a measuring cup combine salt, water, and spices and mix well. This is the brine.

Pack onions into a sterile jar along with any accumulated liquid. Add a weight to keep the onions submerged. Then add brine. The liquid may not cover the onions on day 1. Seal with lid and set in a cool dark place.

The next day, remove lid and top with as much water as necessary to cover the onions. Let stand for 5-7 days, while removing the lid from the jar once a day to let breathe. You will notice bubbles forming as soon as day 2.

Beginning on day 5, you may taste the onions and allow them to continue to ferment until the desired sweet and tangy flavor is reached.

Once fermentation is complete, move onions to the fridge. Eat as desired within 2 months.

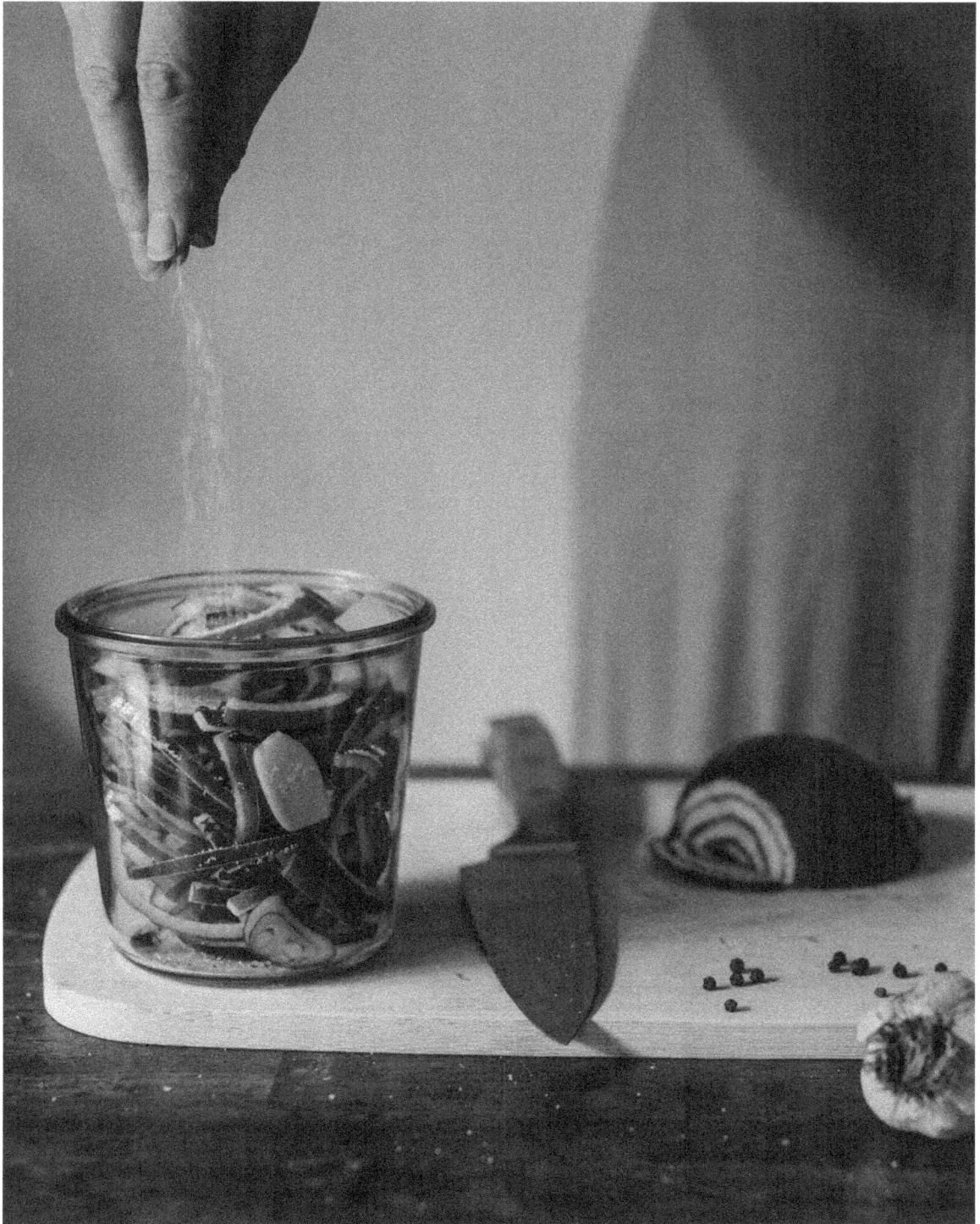

Rosemary Hair Growth Oil

Rosemary has been used to promote hair growth and scalp health for centuries. Known for its ability to improve circulation to the scalp and hair follicles. It also promotes hair growth by providing essential fatty acids and reducing scalp inflammation. It can also balance bacteria to help prevent dandruff. The calming scent has even been shown to reduce stress, which may also lead to hair loss.

Infusing rosemary into beneficial oils like jojoba, argon, or rosehip creates a nourishing blend that can be massaged into the scalp regularly for improved scalp and hair health.

2/3 cup jojoba oil
1/3 cup argon or rosehip oil
1/2 cup dried rosemary
20 drops essential oil of choice (lavender, cedarwood, peppermint)

Infuse oil by using the method described on day 11 or day 20. Strain and store in a sealable glass container, and set in a cool dark place.

To use: Warm oil by placing the glass jar into a bowl of warm water for 20-30 minutes. Add a few drops at a time to the scalp, and massage in as desired. Let sit on the scalp for at least 1 hour or overnight. Wash out normally.

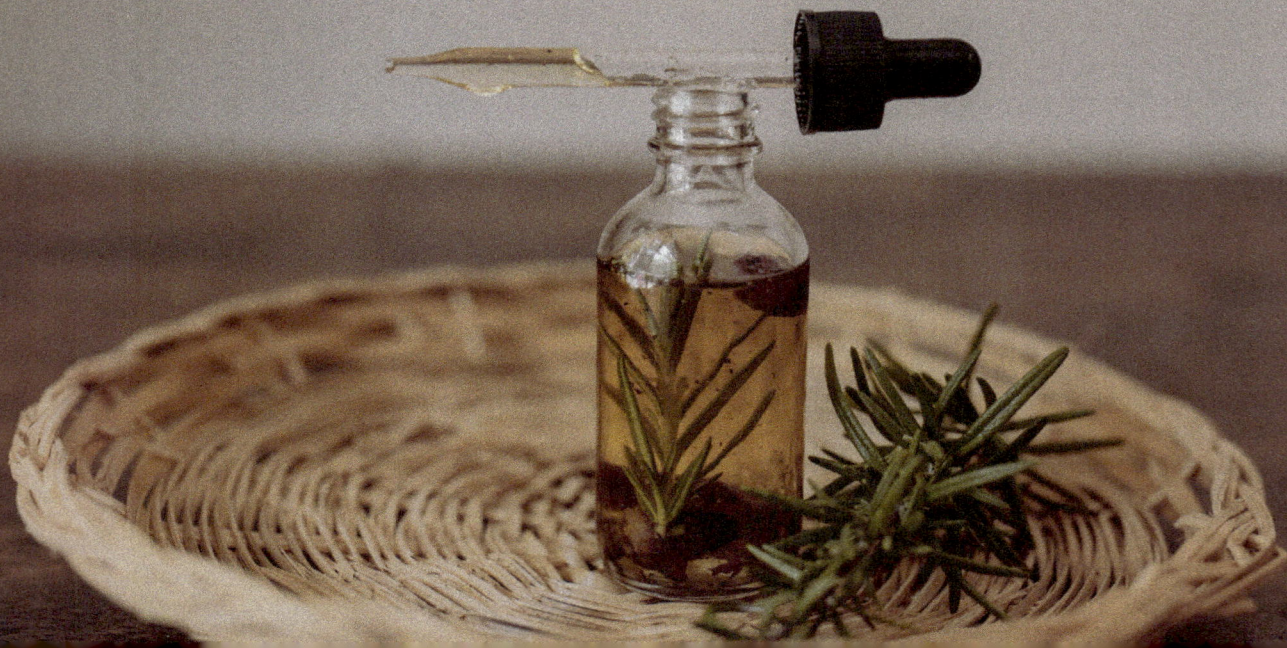

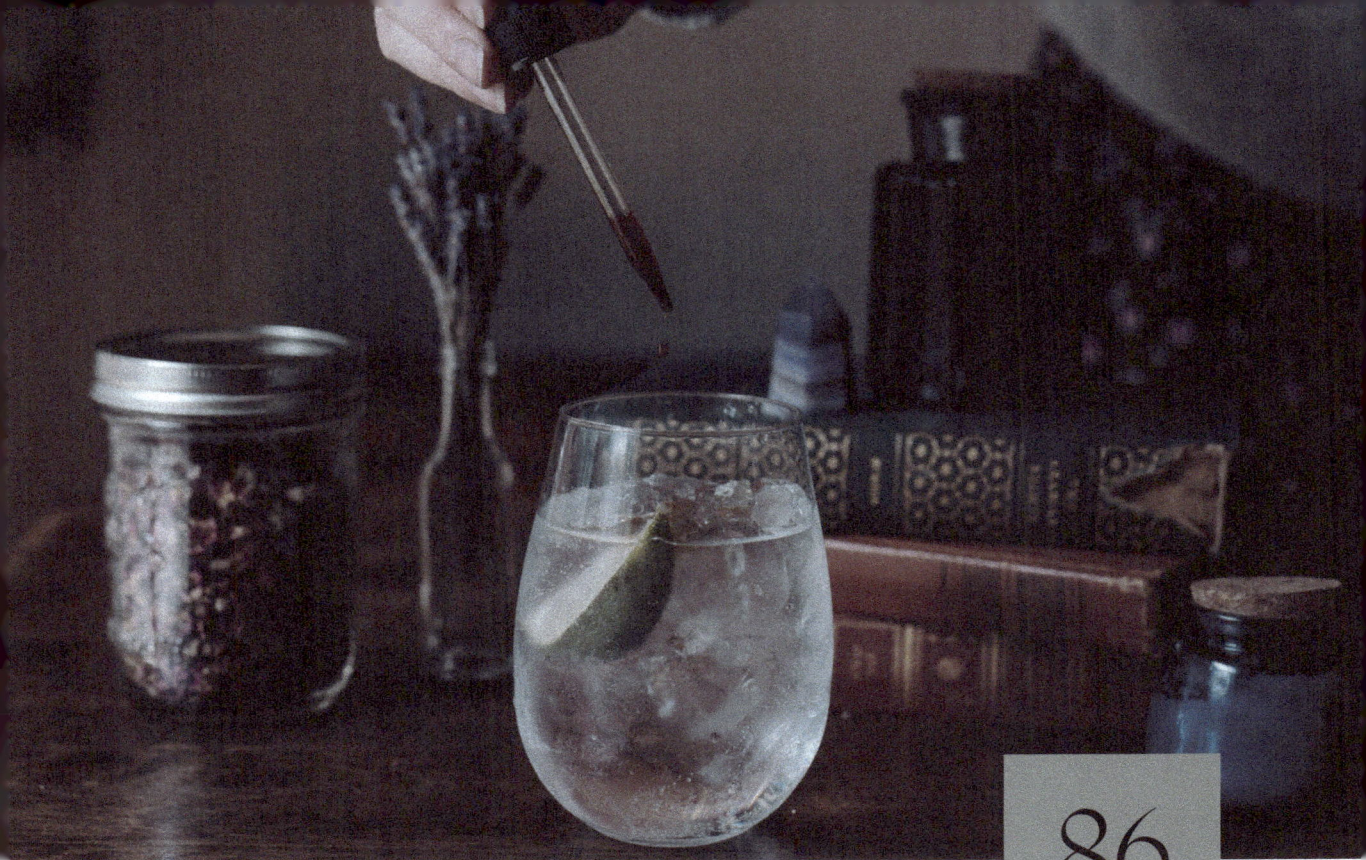

Bitters Soda

The Spiced Bitters tincture made on day 47 has been macerating (soaking or infusing) for 6 weeks, which means it is ready for straining.

Line a fine mesh sieve with a cheesecloth over a large bowl. Pour the infused alcohol and herbs into the cheesecloth. Use the cloth to squeeze out any remaining alcohol from the herbs. Dispose of both the herbs and cheesecloth.

Once strained, store the tincture in a sealable dark glass jar or bottle. Set in a cool dark place for up to one year.

Dosage: 1-3 ml of tincture taken 1-2 times daily, best if at used at least 30 minutes prior to meals.

Bitters soda is a popular way to utilize bitters prior to meals, since this mocktail-style drink retains the bitter flavor along with the added excitement of carbonation.

To make bitters soda, simply add 1-2 droppers of bitters to a glass of seltzer or club soda. Garnish with a citrus wedge and serve cold.

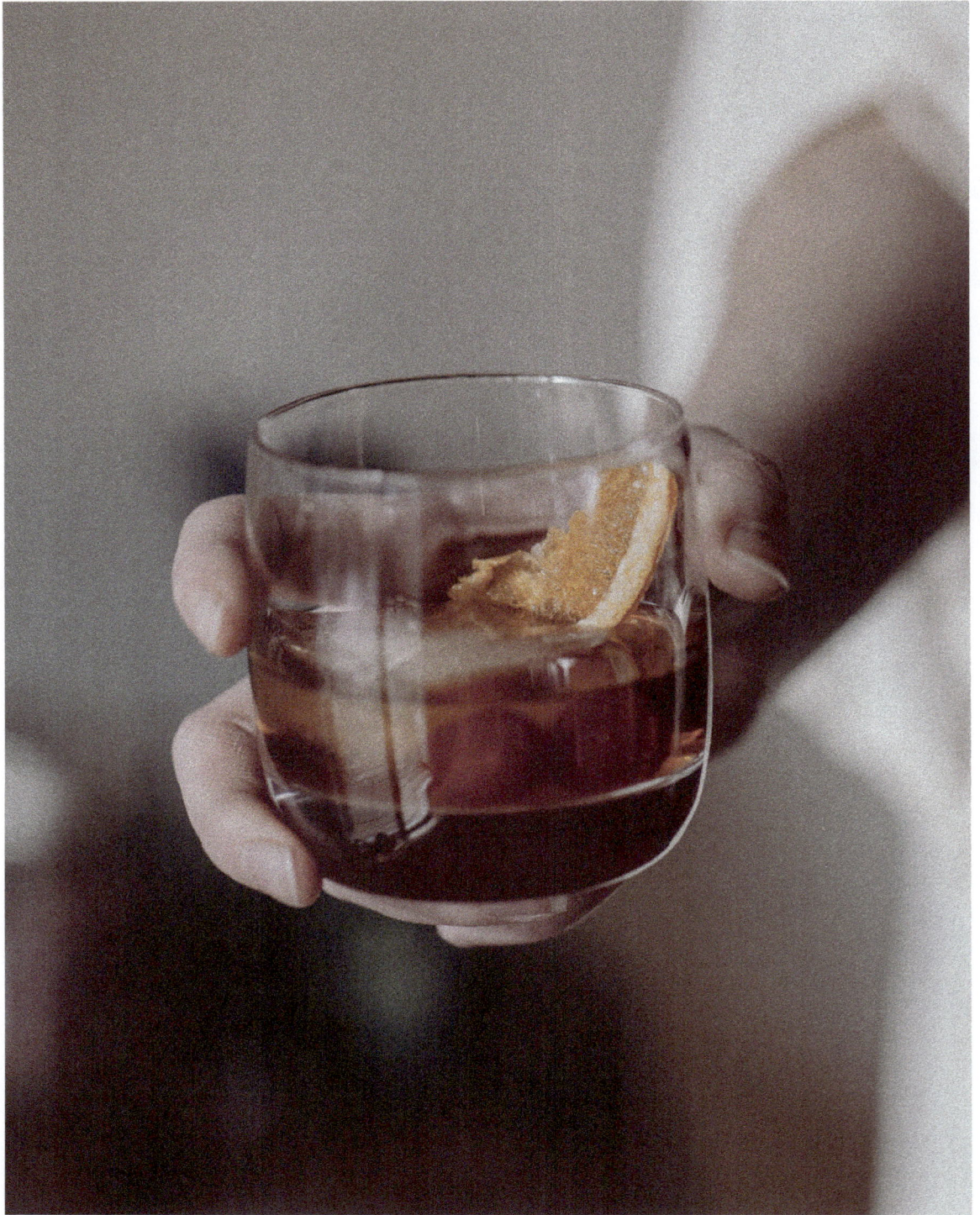

Barley Old Fashioned Mocktail

Old Fashions are a quintessential cocktail with a history that goes back to before fancy cocktails even existed. It is often credited with being the first true cocktail, coming into fashion in the United States in the early 1800's. At that time, it was described simply as sugar, whiskey, and bitters. While there are now many variations, this simple cocktail has fought the test of time and is still a popular drink today.

The great part about this non-alcoholic version, is that it offers many health benefits, including the digestive benefits of bitters. Additionally, barley tea is commonly brewed in East Asian countries and has been touted as aiding in weight loss, blood sugar regulation, digestive support, and improving male fertility. Typically, barley is roasted and produces a dark strong tea that makes a great substitute for whiskey. However, if you are looking for a stronger similarity to a particular whiskey, you can try adding liquid smoke, vanilla, apple cider vinegar, or maple syrup to create a custom whiskey substitute.

Barley Old Fashioned Mocktail

1 bag of barley tea
8 oz hot water
1 sugar cube or dash simple syrup to taste
1 orange slice
1 dropper of bitters
Ice
1 maraschino cherry for garnish

Brew a strong cup of barley tea by combining the tea bag and hot water. Let sit for 20-30 minutes. Let chill for another 20-30 minutes in the fridge. Alternatively, you can make a cold brewed barley tea overnight as described on day 10.

Drop the sugar cube into a rocks glass, along with orange slice and bitters. Muddle lightly.

Add ice cubes as desired and 2 oz of chilled barley tea.

Garnish with cherry and serve.

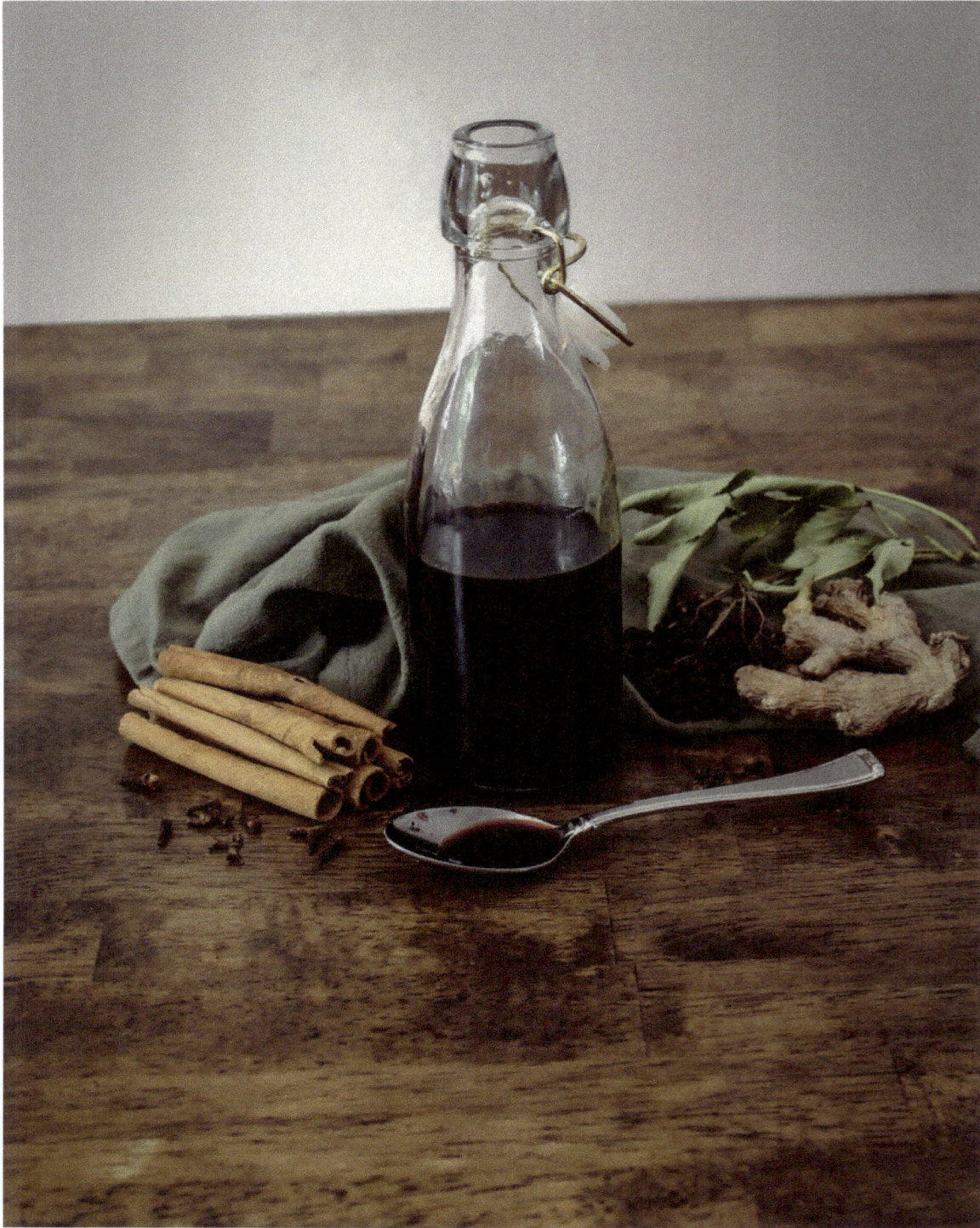

Elderberry Syrup

Elderberry (Sambucus nigra spp.) is an herb that has been used throughout the Americas, Europe, and Northern Asia for centuries. Ancient scholars, like Hippocrates, went so far as to dedicate much of their studies to it. Both the flower and the berry can be used for everything from skin healing, beauty, headache relief, and to improve immunity.

Elderberries are high in antioxidants, anti-inflammatory, alterative, astringent, demulcent, diaphoretic, anti-viral, expectorant, diuretic, vulnerary, and immunostimulant. With these actions, it is easy to see how they can be such a powerful herb in times of cold and flu.

Elderberry Syrup

2 cups dried elderberries
4 cups cold water
2-3 tsp dried ginger root
1 sweet cinnamon stick
2-3 cloves
2 cups raw, local honey (or maple syrup)

Combine all ingredients, except the honey, in a pot and bring to a boil. Reduce heat and allow to simmer 30-40 mins.

Remove from heat and let cool for about 1 hour.

Strain out the solids with a cheesecloth and strainer, making sure to reserve the liquid. Use cheesecloth to squeeze out any remaining liquid. Discard herbs.

Add honey (or maple syrup), stirring until incorporated. You may need to warm slightly, but do not allow the liquid to boil.

Store in an airtight container in the fridge for 4-6 weeks.

To use: For adults, take 1 Tbsp 2x daily when exposed to cold or flu, or when you feel as if a sickness may be coming on.

Traditional Stovetop Chai

Massala Chai has a long history in India, dating back to colonial rule in the mid 1800's. It is a sweetened, milky, and spice-filled black tea. The South Asian people began adding additional spices such as ginger, cardamom, pepper, and cinnamon as a way of protest against the tea foisted on them by the colonizing people.

Massala Chai also contains many beneficial herbs that can help support digestion, reduce gas and bloating, increase nutrient absorption, and improve immune function.

This recipe is an adaptation of the traditional methods of preparing a Massala Chai.

Stove Top Massala Chai

8 oz water
2 cardamom pods, crushed
1/4" slice of fresh ginger
1 tsp whole black peppercorns, crushed
2-3 cloves (optional)
1 tsp cinnamon (optional)
1 Tbsp black tea
4 oz whole milk
1 tsp sugar or more

Bring water, cardamom, ginger, peppercorn, cloves, and cinnamon to a boil over high heat.

Reduce to a simmer and add tea. Cook for 3-5 minutes or until the water is dark brown.

Stir in milk and bring back to a boil. It will bubble and foam. Reduce heat to medium, and cook for 9-10 minutes. The liquid should reduce slightly and turn a tan color.

Stir in sugar. Remove from heat, and strain.

Serve warm.

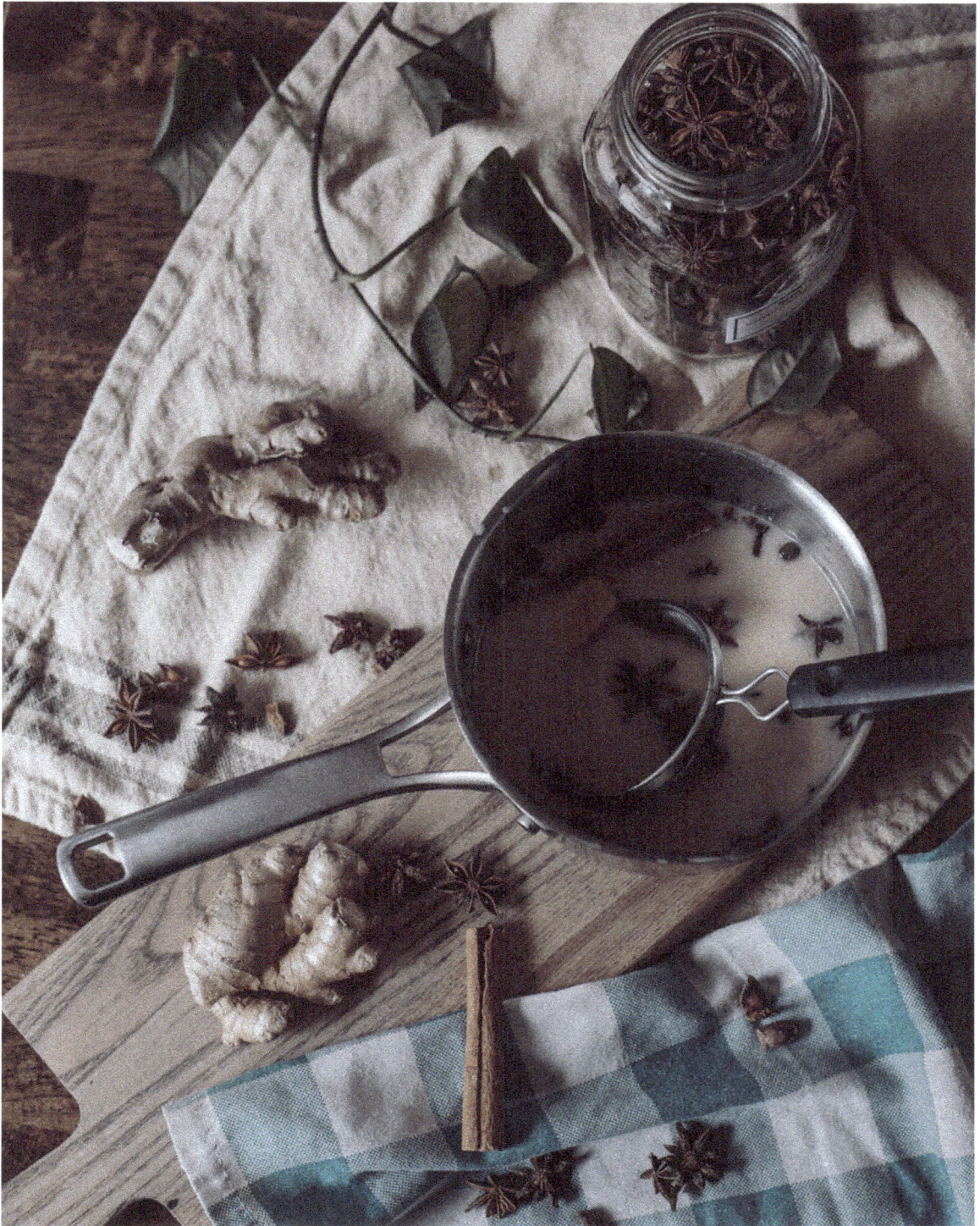

Salad with Fermented Onion Dressing

By now, the fermented onions from day 84 should be ready to eat.

Onions have shown to reduce systemic inflammation, and cellular oxidation,with shallots showing to have the most promise. All varieties of onions, including the red onion (Allium cepa) used for this recipe, are known for promoting strong gut health, immune systems, and aiding in reducing inflammation. Onions are high in quercetin, an antioxidant compound that has been shown to provide protection against cancer, heart disease, and allergies. Incorporating onions, especially fermented onions, into your regular diet can be very beneficial for overall health and longevity.

Salad with Fermented Onion Dressing

1/4 cup fermented onions with juices
2 Tbsp apple cider vinegar
1 Tbsp dijon mustard
3/4 cup extra virgin olive oil
2 tsp salt
¼ tsp black pepper
¼ tsp poppy seeds
2 cups chopped lettuce
1 small cucumber, chopped
2 Tbsp fresh dill, chopped
2 Tbsp fresh cilantro, chopped
1/2 avocado, diced
1 cup chicken, shredded (optional)
1 hard boiled egg, chopped (optional)

In a small bowl, add fermented onions, vinegar, dijon, olive oil, salt, and pepper. Whisk together until well blended. Set aside and prepare the rest of the salad.

In a large serving bowl combine lettuce, cucumber, dill, cilantro, avocado, chicken, and egg. Toss together.

Drizzle with salad dressing and serve.

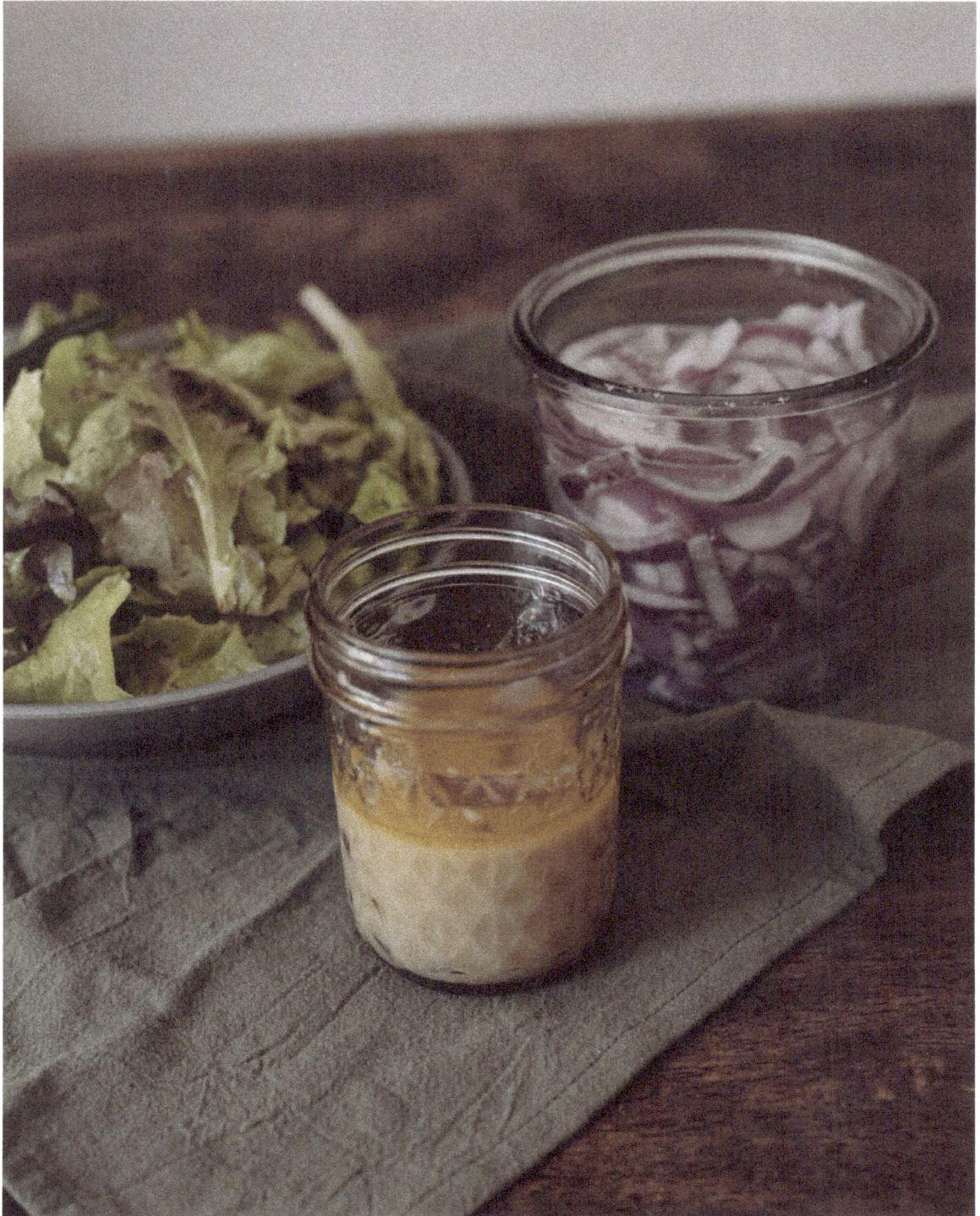

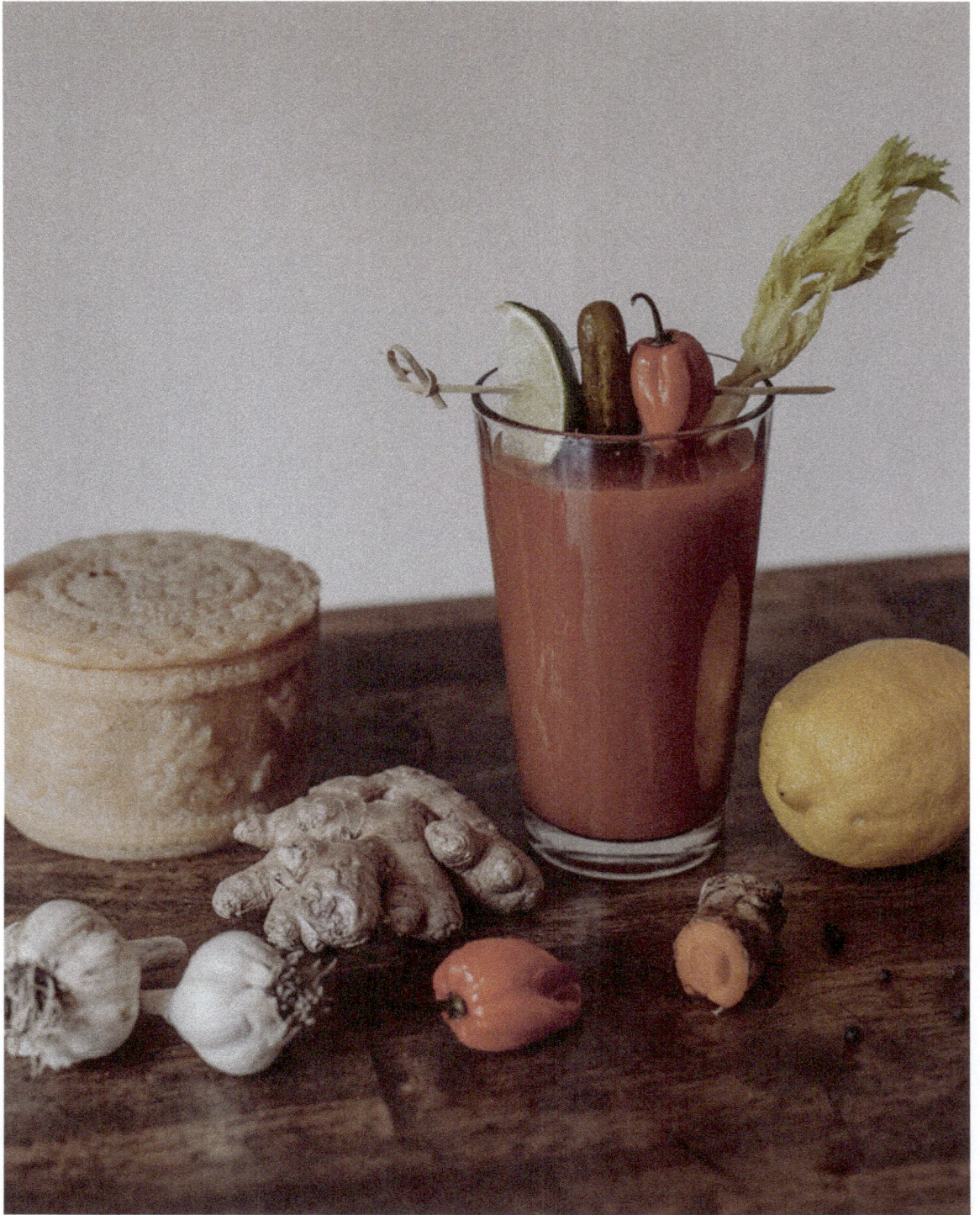

Mock Bloody Mary

The fire cider made on day 67 is ready to decant. To do this, strain out the ingredients through cheesecloth while saving the liquid. Use the cheesecloth to squeeze out additional juice, before discarding or composting. Store the strained liquid in a glass jar in the fridge for up to 6 months.

To use, take 1-2 Tbsp daily when exposed to cold or flu. This can be taken directly or diluted in water. Fire cider can also be used as a spicy salad dressing, marinade, or for a fun mocktail.

Combining the immune boosting benefits of fire cider with the antioxidant and digestive benefits of horseradish, tomato juice, and additional spices make this Mock Bloody Mary a win all around.

Mock Bloody Mary

Celery salt
1 lemon wedge
1 lime wedge
2 oz Fire Cider
4 oz tomato juice
2 tsp prepared horseradish
2 dashes Tabasco sauce (optional)
2 dashes Worcestershire sauce
1 pinch ground black pepper
1 pinch smoked paprika
celery stalk for garnish

Pour some celery salt onto a small plate. Rub the juicy side of the lemon or lime wedge along the lip of a pint glass before rolling the outer edge of the glass in the salt to coat it. Set aside.

Squeeze the lemon and lime into a cocktail shaker before dropping them in.

Add fire cider, tomato juice, horseradish, Tabasco, Worcestershire, black pepper, paprika, and ice. Shake gently.

Strain into the salt-rimmed glass over ice.

Garnish as desired and serve.

92 Create a Blend for Stress and Anxiety

Stress and anxiety are rampant in today's fast-paced world, but luckily there are herbs and practices that can help to combat that. New studies are being conducted every day that confirm what herbalists have known for centuries: herbs are powerful tools used to treat disease and improve mental health, including stress and anxiety.

Use the herbs described below to create a custom blend to combat stress and anxiety. Some important things to consider when creating this kind of blend are how it will be taken; as a tea, tincture, or something else. Utilize herbs that will be beneficial for the method of use you are planning. Refer to additional literature if necessary.

Typically, when looking for herbs that support the body through difficult decisions or feelings, we look for nervines and adaptogens, as well as nutritive herbs.

Nervine Herbs

These types of herbs nourish and support the central nervous system. They can help repair frazzled nerves, and allow the body to relax and recover from stress. The 3 major categories of nervines including nervine relaxants, nervine stimulants, and nervine tonics.

Nervine stimulants engage and excite the sympathetic nervous system. Often, they are used to help with energy and focus, though sometimes they can be overstimulating to sensitive people or already frazzled nerves. These include: coffee, green tea, black tea, cacao, rhodiola, etc.

Nervine relaxants bring a sense of calm and increase activity in the parasympathetic nervous system. They are used to calm the brain and nervous system, helping the muscles relax and release tension. Some of these include: lavender, hops, lemon balm, chamomile, passionflower, skullcap, etc.

Nervine tonics support the nervous system as a whole, and are especially helpful for long term stress or trauma. These types of herbs are not only relaxing to the nervous system, but provide it with the nourishment that it needs to repair and increase resilience. Nervine tonics include: milky oat tops, borage, gotu kola, St. John's wort

Adaptogen Herbs

As discussed throughout this book, adaptogens are herbs that help the body adapt to stress. They tend to have a regulating effect in many ways, including nourishing the adrenal system, supporting the immune system, improving mood, balancing hormones, and fighting fatigue. Some of the most common adaptogens include ashwaganda, reishi, rhodiola, tulsi, ginseng, shisandra, eleuthero, licorice, and maca.

Nutritive Herbs

Nutritive herbs provide the body the with vitamins and minerals necessary for daily functioning. When dealing with stressful situations or big decisions, our bodies tend to burn up vitamins and minerals, so including nutritive herbs can be very helpful. These include raspberry leaf, nettle, oatstraw, clover, alfalfa, dandelion leaf, chickweed, and violet.

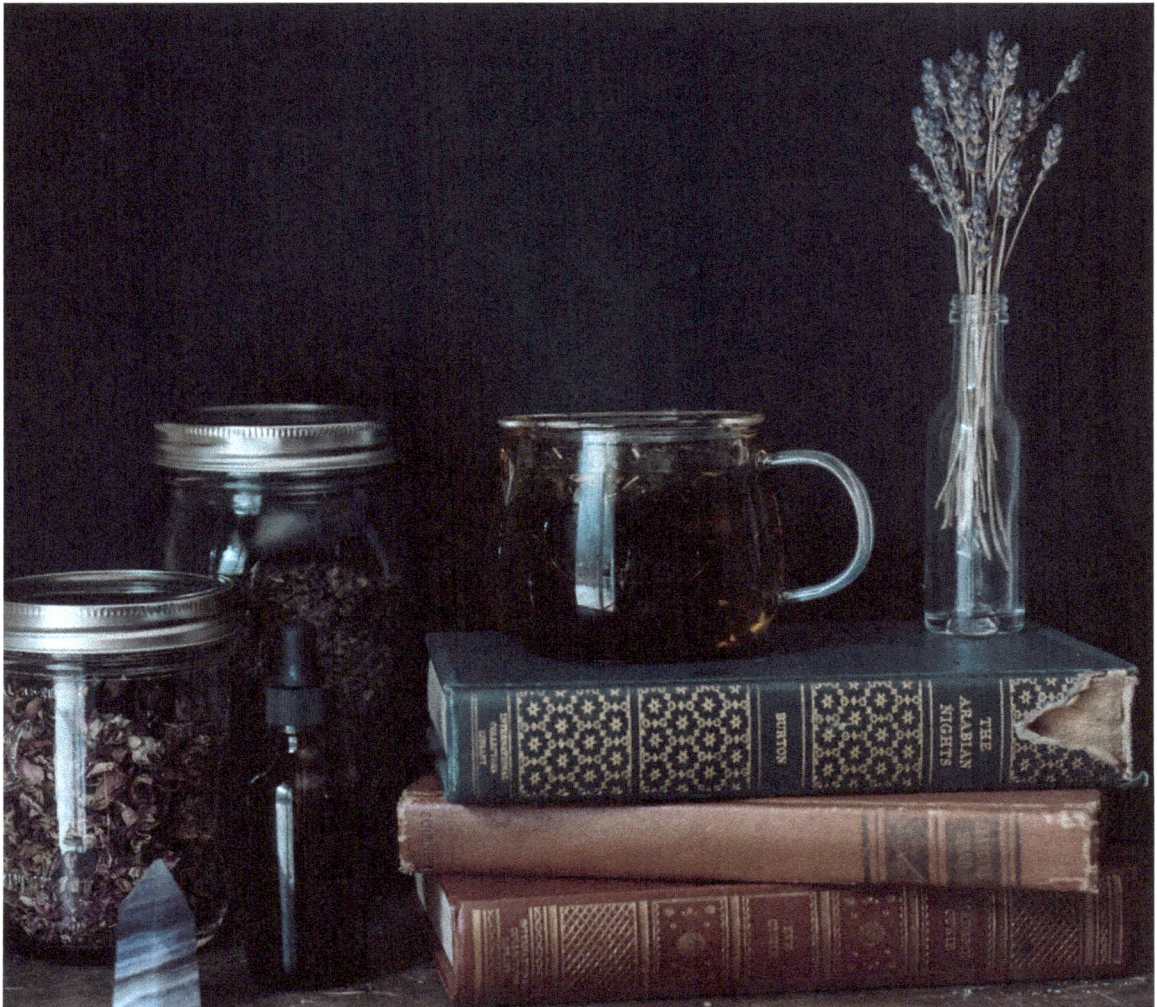

Wound Spray

While the first aid tincture made on day 58 can be used directly on wounds to help staunch bleeding, disinfect, heal bruising, and aid with inflammation; this wound spray is made to disinfect a larger area with ease. Although alcohol – with its disinfectant properties – is used in the mixture, the herbs utilized for this tincture are known for more than this, providing wound healing, blood staunching, promoting cell regeneration, and reducing inflammation.

Yarrow (Achilla millefolium) - Analgesic, antiseptic, anti-inflammatory, promotes healing

Thyme (Thymus vulgaris) - Antiseptic, stimulates wound closing

Lavender (Lavendula angustifolia) - Anti-inflammatory, improves collagen production to promote skin recovery.

Spray Instructions

Use the strained extract to fill a small sterile spray bottle with the strained alcohol tincture and tightly screw on the spray cap.

Mist lightly over affected area immediately after incident, alternatively you could spray the cloth or bandage that is being used to cover the affected area. It may burn slightly when applied as expected with alcohol disinfectants.

Re-apply as needed during re-bandaging.

Discontinue use if irritation occurs.

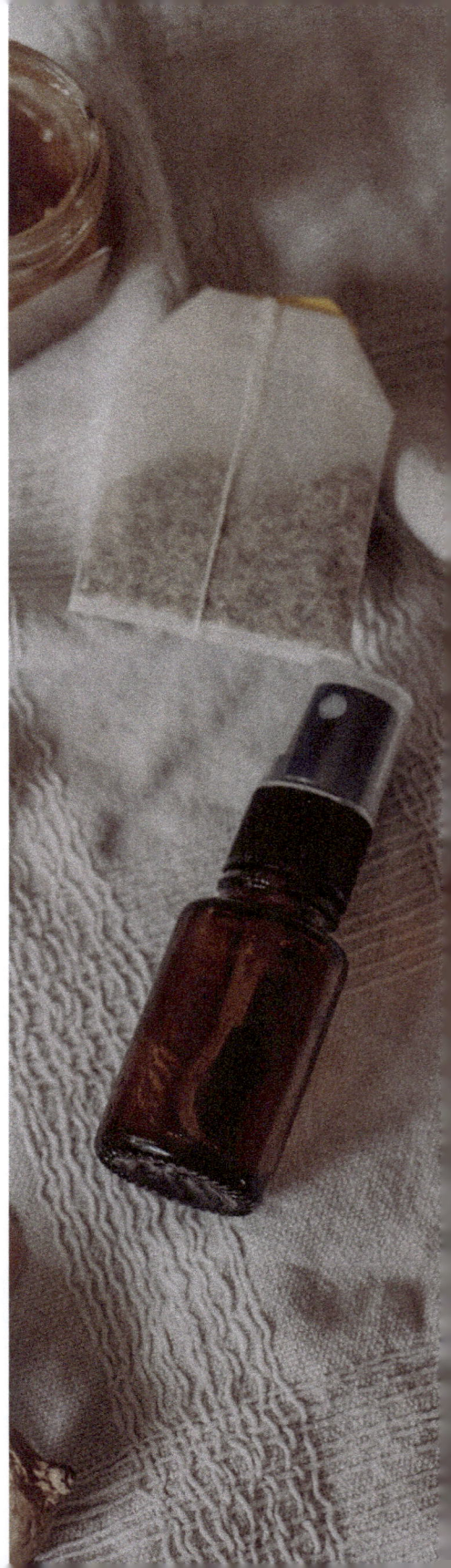

Strain Lemon Balm Glycerite

The Lemon Balm Glycerite made on day 64 has been soaking or macerating for over 4 weeks. At this point in the process, it can be strained and used or stored in a cool dark place.

As discussed on days 4, 59, and 64, Lemon balm (Melissa officinalis) has anti-viral, anti-inflammatory, antiseptic, as well as carminative, mildly sedative, and calming properties. This makes it a great companion for children's care. Not only can it help fight off a virus or bacterial infection, but it can calm a nervous stomach and lull a wee one to sleep. Lemon Balm is even a great companion for calming the nerves before a new adventure or an anxious event.

The mild flavor of lemon balm and the natural sweetness of glycerite makes this an easily palatable medicine for anyone to take.

The dosage for this glycerite range from 4-16ml or 1-2.5 tsp up to 3 times daily. The standard rule of thumb for children's dosage is to use Young's Rule. (Childs Age + 12) / Childs Age = .XX Dosage is .XX the adult dosage

For Example: 4yo child
(4+12)/4 = (16)/4= 0.25
Adult dosage = 1 tsp
Childs dose = 1 tsp x 0.25 = 0.25 tsp

Combine the recommended dosage of lemon balm glycerite with an unsweetened ginger or echinacea tea to help boost the immune system and support healing in the face of cold and flu season.

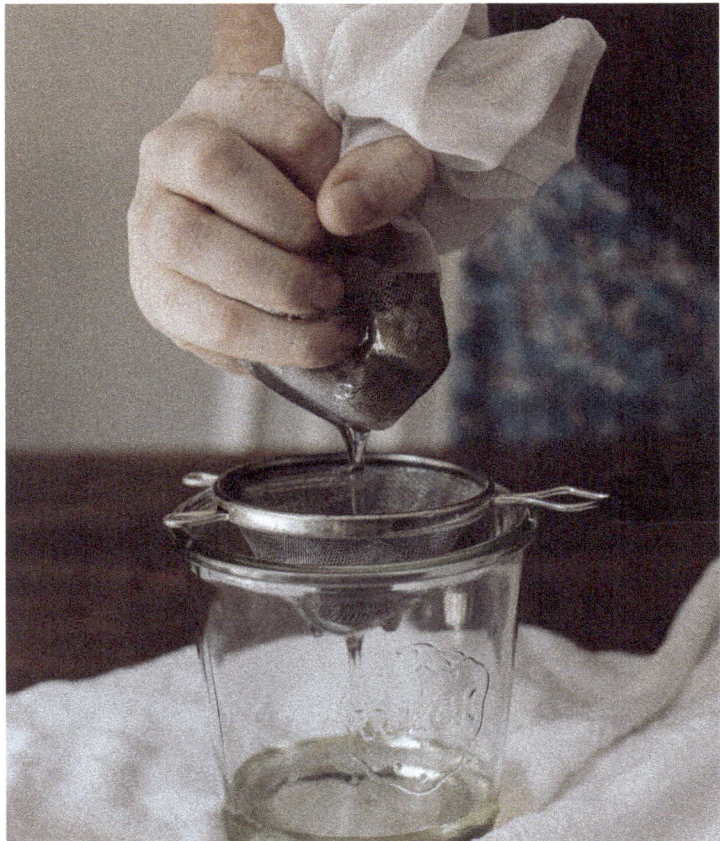

Top Ten

List your 10 favorite herbs and how you typically use them:

Herbal Monographs

An herbal monograph is defined as a document whose purpose is to provide a scientific summary of all data available on the safety and efficacy of an herbal substance or preparation that is intended for medicinal use. They will often also include information on the plants use, history, folklore, and associated legends.

Typically an herbalist compiles their own monographs on the herbs that they use, with information that is tailored to them. Most monographs contain the same basic parts such as a plant's common name, scientific name, plant family, native region, taste, energetics, actions, organ affinity, uses, dosage, precautions, and contraindications. Beyond that-many herbalists will include plant constituents (chemical compounds the plant contains), standard preparations, history, folklore, studies, references, and more. More specifically, an herbalist who has an interest in Traditional Chinese Medicine may choose to include writings, preparations, or history based in that vein, while a South African herbalist may choose to focus on the writings preparations, or history relevant to their area.

It is important to make sure that the information included in a monograph comes from a reputable place, such as a scientific study, high-quality book, or website. It is equally important to distinguish what information is folklore from what is reliable evidence. Many "home remedies" found online may not be as accurate as those from a practicing herbalist or historical text. It can be good to reference several sources on the same topic to draw correlations before administering specific herbs.

When compiling a set of monographs on various herbs into a single document, it is called a Materia Medica. You can begin to create your own Materia Medica by utilizing both the information in this book, reliable herbal references, and your experience with the herbs you have used thus far.

The template for a simple monograph as well as an example monograph are shown on the following pages. To download the template for your own studies go to www.oldwisdomwellness.com/100daysdownloads.

Plant Name . . . .

Scientific Name . . . .

Plant Family . . . .

Parts Used . . . .

Native Region . . . .

Taste . . . .

Energetics . . . .
. . . .

Actions . . . .
. . . .
. . . .

Organ System Affinity . . . .
. . . .

Uses . . . .
. . . .
. . . .
. . . .
. . . .

Dosage . . . .

Precautions . . . .
. . . .

Contradictions . . . .
. . . .
. . . .
. . . .

Plant Name Peppermint

Scientific Name Menta piperita

Plant Family Lamiaceae

Parts Used Aerial Parts, Leaf

Native Region Europe & Middle East

Taste Bold, Stimulating, Cooling

Energetics
Dry/Cooling

Actions
Analgesic (pain relief), Anti-emetic (prevents vomiting), anti-inflammatory, anti-microbial, antioxidant, anti-spasmodic, anti-viral, aromatic, carminative, diaphoretic (induces sweat)

Organ System Affinity
Digestive

Uses
Relaxing effects on smooth muscle and digestive tracts. Nausea, vomiting, spasmodic bowel pain, flatulence, dyspepsia, intestinal colic, diarrhea, ulcerative conditions of the bowels, etc. Can be used as a bitter. Appetite suppressant. Shown to give symptomatic relief in the case of IBS.

Dosage
Infusion: 3-6 g dried leaf/day divided into 2-3 doses; Tincture: 1-2 mL (1:5, 40%) 3x/day

Precautions
May decrease esophageal sphincter pressure, take caution for those with gastroesophageal reflux or hiatal hernia. Also take caution in cases of GI ulcers or significant GI inflammation

Contradictions
Be cautious of use with gallstones.

Begin your Materia Medica

Use your list of 10 favorite herbs from day 95 and create a monograph page for each of them. You can use your own template, or download copies of the one used herein. To download the template for your own studies go to oldwisdomwellness.com/100daysdownloads.

Fill in these monographs as time and information allows, you do not need to finish them all in one day.

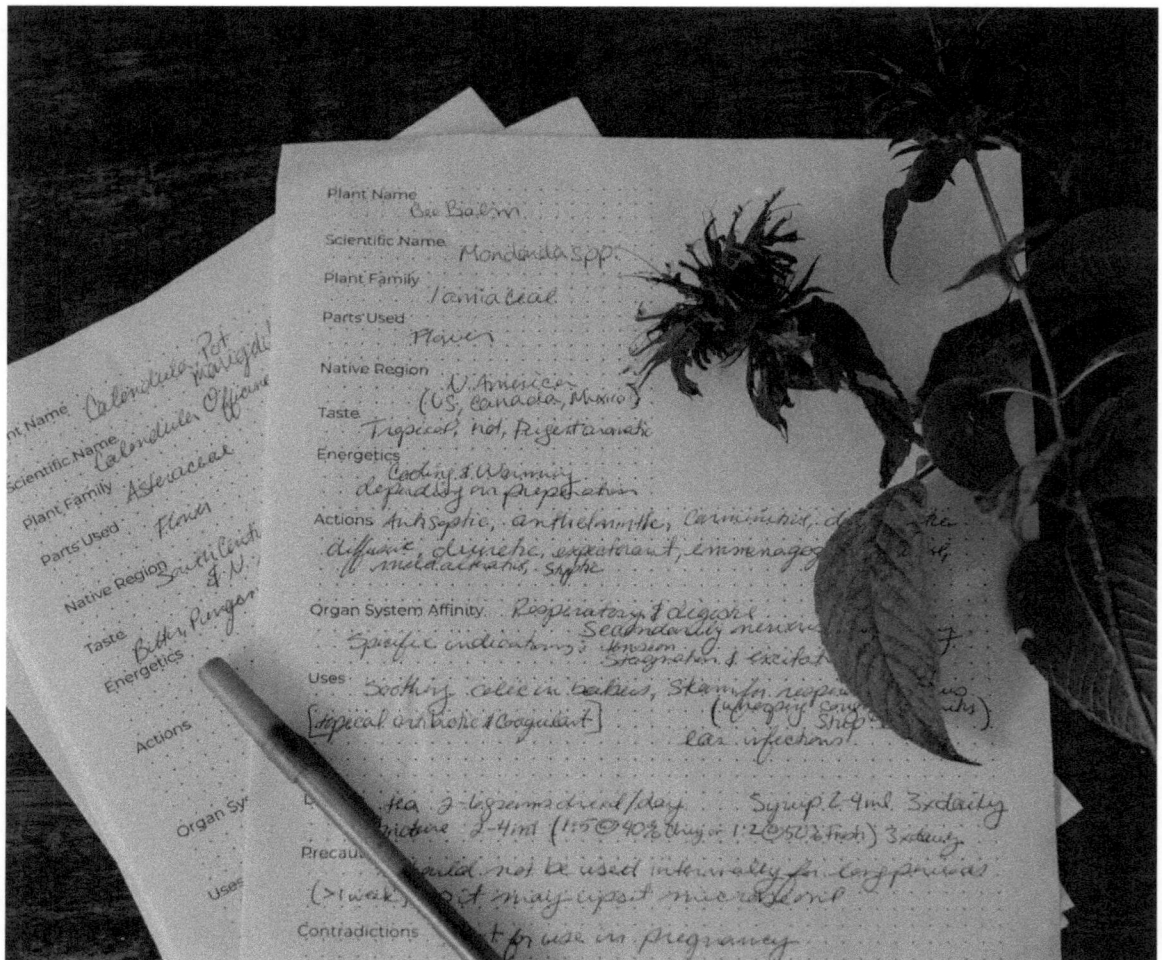

Break it Down

Select a previously made blend and break down it's energetics, taste, and actions.

99

Craft an Herbal First Aid Kit

Over the course of this book we have touched on many different modalities for healing wounds, colds, flu, and other first aid needs. Use that knowledge to create your own herbal first aid kit. Below are some suggestions for herbal components to include:

Honey - Raw honey is a great natural way to cover bug bites, stings, burns, and mild wounds. It is naturally antibiotic, anti-inflammatory, and creates a moist barrier to protect sensitive skin. Raw honey be combined with other items such as styptic powder, wound spray, or tea.

Skin Salve/Oil - Skin salve is a salve that contains skin-healing herbs like the ones used on day 13 and day 23. This comes in handy for cracked hands, rashes, bug bites, and mild wounds. If it's possible that your first aid kit could get left in the heat or sun, you may want to opt for an infused oil instead, as salves are known to melt if they get to warm. Oil is the messier option of the two, but both are powerful allies.

Styptic Powder - Made on day 69, this powder can come in handy to staunch the bleeding of a large wound or cut.

Wound Spray - This spray can be used not only to disinfect wounds, but help remove fungus and bacteria from unwanted places (like athletes foot) and helps to reduce bruising. Find this recipe on Day 54 & 93.

Mint Tea - While mint tea can help with an upset stomach, nausea, and indigestion; it can also help to relax tension and soreness in muscles, headaches, and more. It's always a good idea to have a few extra bags of mint tea on hand.

White Willow Bark - White willow bark has been used for centuries to help reduce pain and inflammation. It is the salicin in white willow bark that was used to develop the main ingredient in modern day aspirin. This item is best if used as a tincture.

Ginger Tea - Similar to mint tea, ginger tea is known to help with nausea and upset stomachs, while also being helpful for pain management

Other items to include: triangular bandage/cloth for a sling or splint, disposable gloves, Gauze pads/roll, band-aids of varying sizes, plastic bags, tweezers, scissors, cold pack, hand sanitizer, thermal blanket, needle & thread.

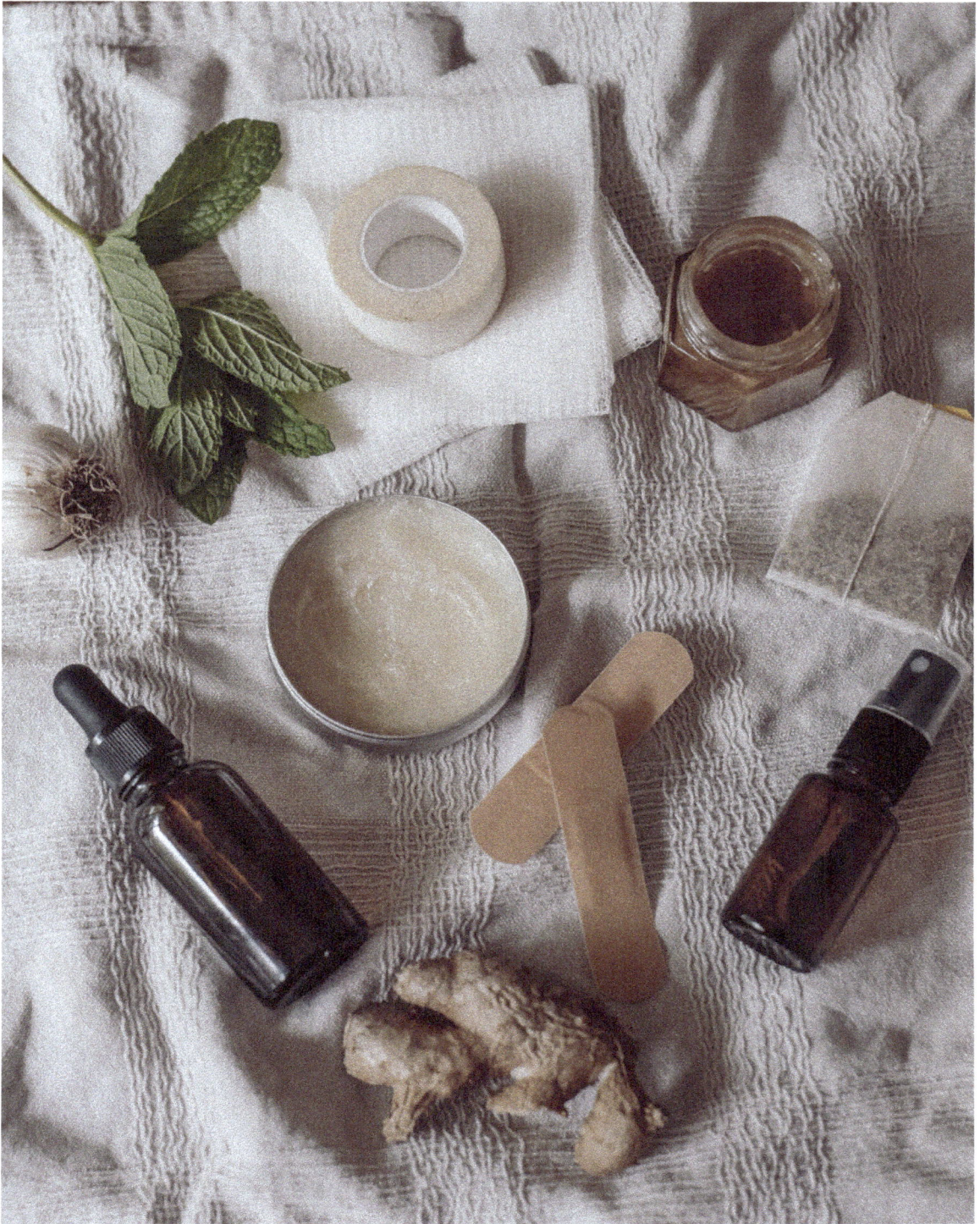

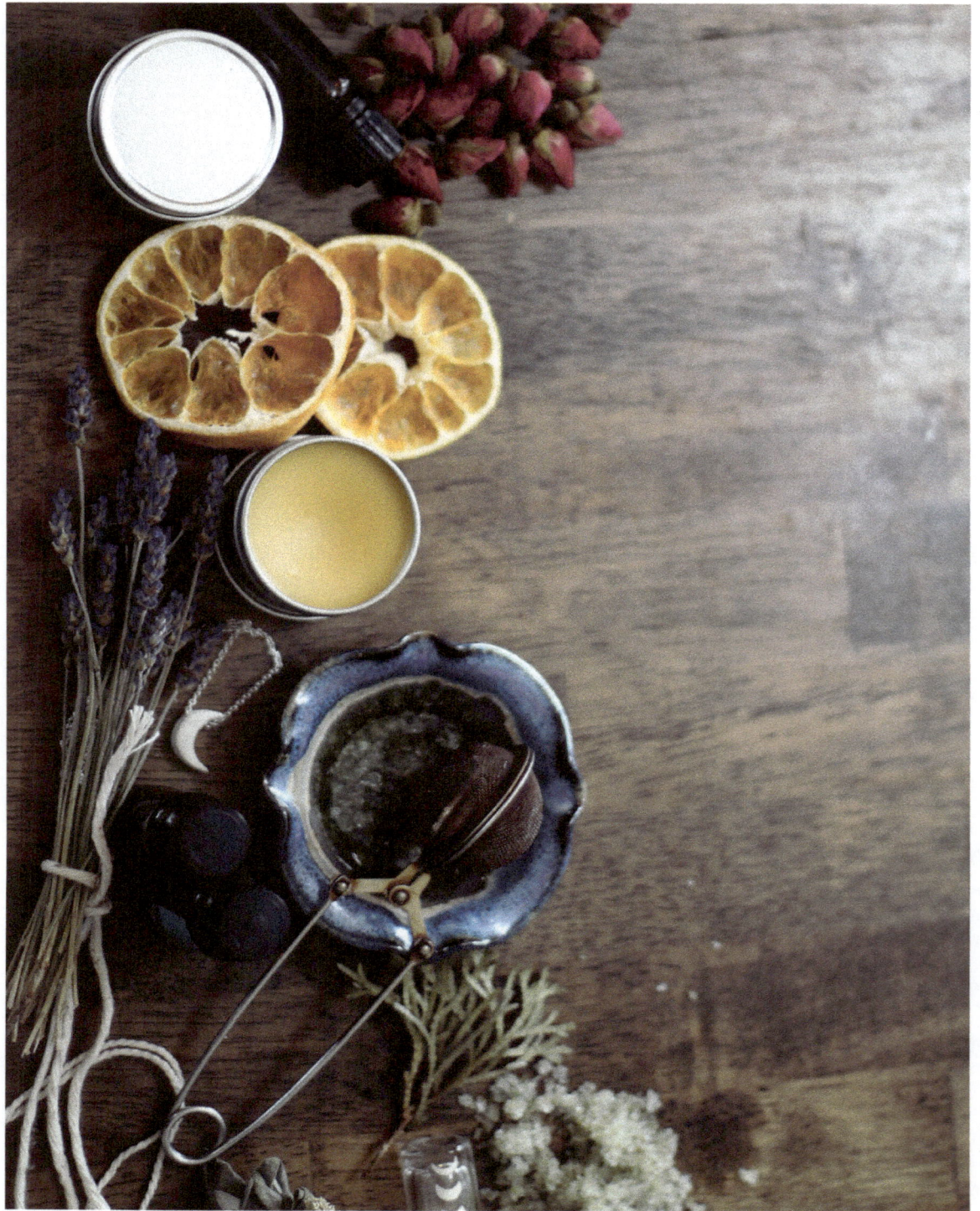

100

Take Stock

In a mere 100 days, this book has covered the foundations of herbalism, touching on the basic concepts, vocabulary, as well as the processes to create healing medicines, cosmetic products, delicious elixirs, and more.

Having gone through this book, you have learned and experimented with many different areas of herbalism. From here, you can take this knowledge into the future in whichever direction you so choose. Whether that is to further study clinical herbalism, maintain a home apothecary, begin a skincare business, or anything in between.

Go back and mark the pages you felt most connected with. Review your journey, everything you have learned, and everything you have yet to learn.

As an herbalist, it is important to have information of various herbs and herbal preparations at your fingertips. While this book is helpful, additional references are necessary. Here is a list of books to help you in furthering your studies:

The Modern Herbal Dispensatory by Thomas Easley & Steven Horne

The Herbal Medicine Makers Handbook by James Green

Holistic Herbal by David Hoffman

Medicinal Herbs: A Beginers Guide by Rosemary Gladstar

Herbal Medicine: From the Heart of the Earth by Sharol Tilgner

A Modern Herbal by Maude Grieve

Herbal Healing for Women by Rosemary Gladstar

Botany in a day by Thomas J. Elpel

For links and additional resources go to www.oldwisdomwellness.com/100daysdownloads

Acknowledgments

First and foremost, thank you to my husband, Eric. Without his support and encouragement, I would never have been able to get this book out into the world. His steadfast strength and guidance have made me the woman and mother I am today.

To my family and friends who supported and held me up in times of doubt, who shouted from the sidelines when I announced my plans to write this book, and when I left my career in search of something more. The confidence you have instilled in me has been invaluable.

Rachel Lanzi, my photographer, was not only able to bring the image in my mind to life but surpass my wildest dreams in her work. Her skill and talent leave me in awe. Find more of her work at thecontentagency.com

My personal unicorn and support system, Taylor MacDougall, who not only took charge of my kids to allow me time to work, but listened to my misgivings and difficulties with the book, business, and life. Additionally, her work on not only beta reading but also editing was invaluable. Find more about her at taylormacdougall.co.

Thank you to all of my Beta readers, who offered wisdom and guidance in developing this final version of the book: Sara Hutcherson of SloBreathworks.com, Melissa Mackinnon, Marcella Hammer, Maria D'Angelico, and Heidi Radko of coreessencecoaching.com.

A special thank you to my patrons and blog readers, past and present. Getting to this point in my business and this book, has been a journey of which even the most anonymous of you have been a part of. I cannot thank you enough for the kind words, corrections, criticisms, and encouragement that I have received from all of you. It has truly helped to mold me into the creator I am today.

A final thank you to our planet for sustaining us, for guiding me, and showing me the joys of nature and all it has to offer.

HERBAL INDEX

HERBAL INDEX CONT...

CATEGORY INDEX

www.ingramcontent.com/pod-product-compliance
Lightning Source LLC
Chambersburg PA
CBHW042336030426
42335CB00028B/3358